Coping with
DISABILITY

Dr Judy Bury, the General Editor of this series, has worked in general practice and family planning for many years. She writes regularly on medical topics, and has a particular interest in self-help approaches to health care.

Coping with
DISABILITY

MILLICENT M. ISHERWOOD

With a Foreword by
Rt. Hon. ALFRED MORRIS M.P.

Chambers

Published by W & R Chambers Ltd Edinburgh

Illustrated by Peter Riches

ISBN 0 550 20512 8

British Library Cataloguing in Publication Data

Isherwood, Millicent
    Coping with disability.
    1. Physically handicapped — Rehabilitation — Great Britain
    I. Title
    362.4'048'0941   HV3024.G7A3
    ISBN 0-550-20512-8

Printed in Great Britain by
Butler & Tanner Ltd, Frome and London

Contents

Foreword

Millicent Isherwood's book maintains the very high standard set by earlier titles in this important series. It is an eminently practical and *readable* guide, long overdue and at once down-to-earth and comprehensive, to how people with disabilities can cope successfully with their handicaps and lead more fulfilling lives.

It seems incredible now, even outrageous, that it was not until 16 years ago that they first had a law they could call their own. In the whole field of social policy, there was no area so utterly neglected, and Millicent Isherwood is right to remind us that there are still people in positions of public authority who drag their feet in implementing the Chronically Sick and Disabled Persons Act.

In Britain today, over 5.5 million people are disabled physically, mentally or sensorily. Yet even that figure tells nothing like the whole story. The mother with a disabled child is involved in the problems of disability, like the child of a disabled mother. Their lives and millions more are profoundly affected by disability in the family. Overwhelmingly, they want those they care for to be a part of, and not apart from society. That, fundamentally, is what this book is all about.

We have here clear and concise information not only about statutory provision and the help voluntary agencies can give, but also on what people with disabilities and their families can do for themselves in tackling the often subtle and complex problems they confront. I know of no more easily readable guide to overcoming the challenges of disabled living, not least those of mobility, social relationships, employment and recreation.

I hope this book will be widely read in the caring professions as well as by disabled people and their families. It will be invaluable also to decision-makers and those who plan the provision of statutory and voluntary help. By reading *Coping with Disability*, they will have an experienced and intelligent consumer's guide to the effectiveness of their work. At the same time it may remind them of the wisdom of Oscar Wilde's wry inference when he said, after the first night of one of his plays, that the play was a great success but the audience a failure.

All too often people with disabilities are expected to be passive and dependent in accepting what others decide is best for them. Happily, there is nothing even remotely submissive in

Millicent Isherwood's approach. From long first-hand experience of triumphing over handicap, she offers a deep insight into all the problems of disabled living and conveys the unambiguous message that disabled people are entitled to the same rights as everyone else. In following her example and advice, they will find that much more control over their own future can be theirs for the taking.

The Rt Hon Alfred Morris PC MA MP
House of Commons, July 1986

1. Introduction

This book is a series of signposts pointing to helpful agencies, special aids, tactics and strategies. There may be new ideas or new perspectives for old campaigners as well as for the recently disabled. There are so many forms of disability that what helps one person may not help another. The character and personality of the victim and of the carer (if there is a carer) are major forces in coping with disability and what makes sense for one person will not perhaps succeed for another.

I propose this definition of disability—it is a weakness or failure of some working part of the body or head. Great effort is needed to do essential things which most people accomplish easily; some functions may be impossible. Walking, talking, seeing, hearing, breathing, eating, communicating, understanding may be impaired or impossible without special aids. This book is particularly for those who have mobility problems, and for their carers.

I was 95% disabled by polio in 1947 at the age of 22. Since then disabled people have emerged into the outside world, have sought (with some success) access to public buildings, jobs, travel facilities on planes, trains and buses. The mobility allowance is enormously enabling. It is given in cases of extensive paralysis, or when two legs have been amputated, one above the knee. You will no doubt be told of people who were given a free car and a mobility allowance after breaking a leg but you can safely deny this!

There is a tendency for the general public to overestimate what is available for the disabled and sometimes resentment is felt by the able-bodied because of this. For example, I have tried three times unsuccessfully to park at Tarn Hows in the new, clearly-labelled park for disabled drivers supplied by the

National Trust. The cars there were never all driven by disabled drivers. As one car-driver came back from her walk she looked at my orange disc and said to her friend, 'I have to take pills for the rest of my life but no-one gives me a disc for my car'. I hope her car enjoyed the view.

Since the Alfred Morris Act of Parliament made it a legal requirement that public buildings should provide access for disabled people, life has become richer, but it is surprising how many responsible bodies ignore the law. When I attended my first meeting of the County Council Social Services Committee there were some red faces at the County Hall which had no lift (14 years after the Act had been passed). Some of the red faces belonged to the junior officers and porters who had to carry me up and down stairs. It is still not assumed that disabled people will enter government although often they are articulate. They often have unused energies because of the limitations imposed by their disability. There is a theory that certain types of personality are found to develop certain types of illness. Whether the illness's restraints and difficulties shape the personality or not, I don't know. An interesting area to research, perhaps—useless, but interesting!

When stricken we are numb, then enraged, then afraid. We 'rage, rage against the dying of the light'. The emotions are strong, violent and for a time overwhelming. You learn to channel them, to use them, to make them the steam that drives the engine of your life. You have to do this in your own way and at your own speed. Sharing violent emotion can extend and double it. Steam has no force unless it is contained and directed. It is good to let off steam occasionally, but not too often. You lose power that you need and you can scald other people. There are many stages of development, some very painful and some very rewarding, but it is a journey and you pass on.

Sometimes *carers* face the problem first. They may be informed when the victim is too young or too ill to know. Never take over the thinking or the suffering or the decision-making of the disabled person. You do not have that right and it will impair your functioning as carer and enabler. You will feel the need to share the frustration and the suffering but as a carer you will have suffering and frustration of your own, of a different kind, from which you cannot escape. Save your endurance for that. Don't let anyone do your thinking for you or make decisions for you. There is within each of us a core of being which feels strongly what is right for us. Beware how you try to think, or make decisions, for others. Often those who are nearest and dearest to us make totally wrong assessments of our feelings, reactions and stamina under stress. 'In the presence of trouble some people buy crutches and others grow wings'. It is not easy to predict which people will do which. Both disabled people and carers must keep the right to make their own decisions and to make their own mistakes. Those who never make mistakes never make anything. It's a very important part of living and growing.

Whether the onset of disability is sudden or gradual, end-stopped or on-going, there is always a moment of impact, a sudden perception for victims and carers which is devastating. The effect cannot be considered in isolation. So much depends on the spirit, the skills, the temperament and (very important) the financial resources of those affected. Storm-tossed and pilotless on an ocean of darkness, those most wanting to help are often least able to do so. Some consultants are good judges of how much the stricken can take in and they speak clearly in layman's terms. Some use technical language and make reference to research and are disturbed by their inability to cure. Most general practitioners are used to picking up the pieces, answering the questions, repeating medical details when you are ready to understand and remember them. The GP sees the family as a whole and the doctor with listening ears will know what help to offer and when to offer it.

Help is not necessarily where you expect it to be. Some friends ask awkward questions, others do your ironing while you talk. Some pick up your laundry and take it home to do it for you. They may sympathise, make a meal for you and yours, weep, be jolly and bracing and all can be mixed blessings. You will come across help unexpectedly from unlikely sources. New friends will appear. Different pilots are needed for different stretches of the journey. If some kind of help comes when you are not ready for it and you can't accept it or make use of it, then however good it is, it is useless to you. Remember this when you try to help others. You will use helpers on the way and then your paths will diverge.

You in your turn will come across people who need the help that only you can give. Remember to be understanding, not offended, if they are at a stage when they can't accept or use your help. If they do use your help don't cling to them afterwards or expect them to cling to you. Sometimes help is offered ineptly or brusquely or tactlessly. Be understanding of the difficulties of those who feel for you and who want to help but don't know how best to do so. Remember too that it is within your power to demand help in a way that makes it difficult or impossible to refuse. Beware! It's not the fault of the able-bodied that you are disabled. Nor is it yours, everyone knows that. But if you become too demanding you will perhaps find that there are fewer people around you to be asked.

Life as a disabled person is like fell-walking. (I wrote this in the Lake District at Castlerigg Stone Circle). Rising, descending, striding and stumbling in mist and rain or sunshine and steam, high peaks and low troughs with hard falls and splendid views after long struggle, wearying and breathtaking, life's taste-buds are assaulted by more of the bitter and more of the sweet than the average human being experiences. One needs to be, and hopefully one becomes, more alert and more sensitive.

'Cures'

A very important matter, 'cures'. You cannot demand, and money cannot buy, cures that do not exist. This is a very important crossroad on the journey forward. You become the natural prey of purveyors of 'cures' brought about by diet, climate, herbs, faith, exercises, ointment, jewellery, new philosophies.

The most *distressing* part of this is that many purveyors are genuine in their desire to help. They believe in what they offer.

The most *difficult* part of this is that one should be open-minded, remembering the scorn that was heaped upon antisepsis measures when they were new.

The most *dangerous* part of this, for disabled people and carers, is that the offers tried, the measures pursued, the hopes raised, delay the most essential part of coping with disability successfully. This essential act is to face it, examine it, explore it, come to terms with it. Others have. You can. If at present you are at the beginning of this journey you will feel that you are not going to succeed. But you will.

You need the strength to change the things that must be changed; the courage to accept the things that cannot be changed; and, above all, the wisdom to know the difference.

Summon all your strength to do all you can and this includes doing the impossible. Muster every atom of willpower to forget forever what you will never be able to do again. Use all wit, wiles, intelligence, ingenuity, inventiveness and cunning (your own and other people's) to make certain what is and what is not possible.

If in this book I misfire, forgive me. If you are not ready for some of the advice, wait and see. If anecdotes annoy, skip them! If what I say is helpful it makes use of some of my past pain in a positive way. You won't have exactly my problems but strategies can be adapted.

2. Who Cares?

Your doctor, as well as being an encyclopaedia of treatments, is your introduction to a series of invaluable services. Ask him or her what he/she thinks you need. You may benefit from social workers, occupational therapists, health visitors, home nursing, home helps, meals-on-wheels, visiting a day-centre or a chiropody service. Public libraries often run a home-visiting service, though provisions vary in different areas.

Electricity and Gas and Solid Fuel have information about their facilities and special equipment. In the case of gas appliances there are free safety checks though not free repairs.

Social Services

Social services will visit you, if asked to do so, to assess the help you need. They will tell you of the benefits to which you may be entitled and will organise an occupational therapist to advise you on aids, house-adaptation, applying for the necessary planning permission and for financial help. Occupational therapists have an invaluable store of information, ideas, knowledge of procedures and dates of meetings when planning applications are processed. (As these are usually held monthly you can save four weeks' waiting by meeting the deadline).

The Department of Health and Social Security

The DHSS post leaflets to you about available benefits if you phone or write to them. Public libraries also stock the leaflets. You may possibly be entitled to a pension, invalidity benefit, attendance allowance, supplementary benefit, help with special costs of diet, heating, laundry. This is a very complicated area regularly revised by acts of Parliament. The whole provision needs streamlining and the staff of the DHSS are under great strain because of the unnecessary complications of making this messy collection of antique legislation clear to the public and fair to those who should benefit. They are also short-staffed. Most of the staff are kind and helpful to those in need, but remember their problems! If you are housebound and explain your need to see someone, a member of the DHSS staff will call,but because of staff shortages you may have a long wait.

Physiotherapy

The physiotherapy department of the nearest hospital will loan walking aids if you need them. Physiotherapists will also show carers how to move and lift safely as well as showing how patient and carer can help each other. They know the body's mechanism better than anyone and can make sure you make best use of whatever movement you still have. They are also most experienced in how long a time improvement can go on after you have had any disabling illness.

Wheelchairs and artificial limbs are supplied through Appliance Centres and aids for seeing and hearing through the out-patients departments of hospitals.

Age Concern

This organisation (in the phone directory) is nationwide and mainly voluntary although there is a small number of paid helpers. Services vary from area to area but usually include advice on benefits, 'pop-in' refreshment rooms serving tea and coffee and light meals, luncheon clubs for limited numbers, occasionally a minibus which may take one or two wheelchairs. As the name of the organisation suggests, this provision is for people over 60 years of age. You may be able to help here, manning a telephone perhaps.

British Red Cross

The BRC (in the phone directory) is worldwide, non-sectarian, and exists to help those who are ill or disabled. It is a voluntary organisation and what it provides depends on how many volunteers it has in the area. Trolley shops and library trolleys are run in hospitals and old people's homes. Medical aids are loaned free of charge, but crutches are not. Welfare visiting of old people is undertaken. In dire emergencies night-sitting might be arranged for a short time. Money is always needed and fund-raising is important as well as much appreciated.

Women's Royal Voluntary Service

This is nationwide and the services provided in an area depend on how many volunteers there are. The aim of the WRVS is to give help in the community. Clubs, meeting weekly, are organised for the elderly and for the disabled. Meals-on-wheels and luncheon clubs provide main meals at nominal cost and are so popular that the advice of Social Services is often sought to decide who should benefit. Books-on-wheels are organised in homes for the elderly and in some hospitals in consultation with the Red Cross (so that there is no double provision). You may be able to help here, if the office is accessible. If all members are involved in the work, the office phone is not manned all the time.

Disablement Resettlement Officer

This person is to be found in every Job Centre. To contact the DRO look up Manpower Services Commission in the phone book. Smaller Job Centres may only have the DRO on duty part-time but you will always be told when the DRO is there, and your enquiry will be followed up. If you are interested in the Professional and Executive Department they use the services of the Job Centre DRO who has at his/her disposal professional help with assessment and, if advisable, retraining. All disabled applicants are seen, medical reports are studied, and a second interview is arranged to discuss employment possibilities.

Societies

National societies associated with particular diseases have grown up to finance research and disseminate knowledge. These societies are invaluable. No general hospital and no general practitioner has the opportunity to amass the depth and breadth of experience which these specialist groups have. I could never have coped with my mother's diabetes, which developed when she was 79 and not fit to cope herself, without the British Diabetic Association. I am forever grateful to the hospital ward sister who gave me the address saying 'They're ever so much better than we are about diet'. Their magazine *Balance* is a splendid read for anyone, diabetic or not.

If you can't bear the thought, and many can't, of going among a group of people who have nothing in common but a handicap, give financial support and help yourself by buying all the leaflets and magazines they supply.

When I was young and newly disabled I hated going among disabled people. It seemed that I was agreeing with what had happened to me, and I wanted to fight it, ignore it, be as normal as possible. Individuals feel very strongly in this area. Yet it is wise to try something before rejecting it as wrong for you. Although there is no logical reason why you should have an affinity with people who have the same medical problem, you may find good friends and good practical ideas of the kind books don't give. The sharing of experience is unique, invaluable, and may be a blessing to carers if not to victims. There is an address list of many of these societies in the Appendix of this book. If there is one you need which we have not listed, ask Social Services, the Public Library Reference department, the Citizens Advice Bureau, or your doctor.

If you want to get involved, the most useful exercise is to raise money—research needs lots of it. Organise a coffee-morning or bring-and-buy sale at your own house. Make posters to advertise events and persuade friends and local shops to display them in their windows. Make toys, toffee, legwarmers, mittens, gay waistcoats, biscuits and buns. These things give you people-contact and a goal to aim for. If you can inspire enough people to make things, the quickest way to sell them is by hiring a stall for a day in the nearest market. Cold, usually, in our climate but an exhilarating experience.

3. How Old Are You?

The pre-school child is portable. The young disabled need care and are dependent as are all young children. The school-age child is 'knocked into shape' by a society which decides what that shape should be. We all remember this, at times painful, experience when sometimes we hurt others because we are hurt ourselves. 'Children can be cruel' it is said, and all parents know the particular pain which comes from seeing their child face rejection in some form. As the young move further from the family circle some of their peers are supportive and some are destructive. Friendships form when they are allowed to do so but no child has autonomy and adults can and do interfere. Since all children are thus imposed on, the disabled child is not yet fully aware of the limitations which will be imposed on it by society. Accepting some restrictions and fighting against others is a step towards independence which will be made healthily if the carer gets it right. Support is needed *but sympathy may not always be supportive.*

The Adolescent

The adolescent is self-preoccupied. The peer group is all-important to the teenager. (The 'teenager' was invented in the 1950s, remember). It is against the peer group that the adolescent measures him/herself. Appearance is all-important (yes!) and experiments in clothes, hairstyles, manners, language and music are made which leave adults gasping. This is the intention; this is a world in which the adult has no place. If adolescents argue, emotion is aroused out of all proportion to the importance of the subject under discussion. The individual is fighting to be free to develop, free to think, free of society's clutches. Society seems in need of an overhaul. This is the age of dire despair, delirious delight and of deafness. The chief adolescent complaint is, 'They all shout at me', (teachers, parents). The pop music is turned ever louder to shut out the adult instructions, advice, reminiscences. The next main adolescent complaint is, 'They're always on about when they were my age—I can't help that, that was centuries ago'. Quite right. Now, more than at any other age, it is painful to be an outsider. This is the hardest time for anybody but it is especially hard for the disabled adolescent. A teenager can descend into despair if the nose is the wrong shape or if the hair is too curly or too straight. Hell gapes in front of the disabled teenager. 'Will I ever marry? Will I ever have children?' The answer must always be, 'Possibly. And anyone who marries you will be special and brave and well worth marrying'.

Adolescent rebellion is seen as a necessary part of human development in the latter part of the twentieth century. I have never forgotten the cry of one mother, 'Why oh why is my daughter in the throes of adolescent rebellion when my mother's going senile and I'm in the menopause?' So ponder the predicament of the disabled adolescent who may be dependent for regularly-recurring physical attention on the adults against whom rebellion is usually directed. Don't think, as a carer, that if you've evaded trouble all is well. It is possible that it may surface later or later still and be harder to handle. Or there may be an increased dependency and a regression to childlike behaviour which is bad for all concerned. This can hold the seeds of tragedy for the time when the carer may be ill or old. Be a welcoming host for the peer group. Leave them alone with plenty of soft drinks and pop records to be young together. Let friendships develop. Take risks. Give opportunities for young friends to take over some of your carer duties. See if it is possible for outings to be arranged without you going along. There is a vast untapped reservoir of caringness and dedication in young people. They care about each other more than most adults realise. As adult commitments pile up, time becomes precious and other things crowd out the opportunities to care in the same way. Make hay in the summertime. When autumn comes there will be happy memories.

Adolescence is the time when plans are made for the future, for after-school life. Plans may be shattered by economic recession, exam failure, family break-up, being rejected after interview, but disabled people have fewer options to begin with. Endless steps and scattered buildings in universities and colleges of further and higher education are major impediments to advanced education. Accommodation difficulties away from home are another. The Open University is a blessing. The aim should be to get as much further education as possible. Disabled people need to be better qualified than the rest to get to the same end, an interview.

There is a lot of advice in print about how to succeed in interviews and the disabled person has only one extra problem. That is to convince the panel of interviewers that you are reliable and that if your vehicle lets you down you have alternative transport near at hand. 'We always use the taxi-firm in the next street', is a better bet than 'my dad', I feel.

The Newly Adult

This is the pre-responsibility fun-time. There are no large claims on your cash and you can do what you wish with what you earn. You are freer than you ever have been or will be. If disability strikes or starts to nibble now, you have some advantages. You have qualified for work, have had some work experience, exist as a contributing member of the Health Service and have a number to prove it. You have a lifestyle which gives you a base from which to make plans. You may get back to work or train for different work. You may adapt your house or move to a different kind of accommodation. If it is necessary you will be given help in the house; if you're earning you will be able to pay for help. You may have caring relatives but future plans must allow for the aging and death of older relatives. You are your own life-force and architect and the only advice you need is not to move too quickly to a solution. It is sad to spend money and energy on detailed and perfect house adaptation and then find you are offered promotion—in another part of the country. The main thing to remember is that money is a great enabler. If it is at all possible, get paid employment, acquire money however much effort it takes. You need efficient heat, a very comfortable bed, domestic help, a car and perhaps a wheelchair or electronic aids. Although you can get some of these things from the DHSS life is easier if you can choose and buy whatever you think you need. The joy of living alone is that you can make yourself comfortable and efficiently self-supporting in your own home with whatever *you* decide is life-enhancing.

The Responsible Adult

This is the time when anything that affects you probably affects a family too. You may have gathered responsibility for a partner, children, aging parents, a mortgage, a car, as well as a heavy work-load with high stress. This is a case for thorough family consultation. Being disabled puts other worries in their place. First, consider the medical advice. Will work be possible for the foreseeable future? For a limited time? Or not at all?

Then consider financial matters. Can you get a capital sum to give some income? There may be compensation if you had an accident, or some insurance if you had a policy, or a lump sum if you have to retire early. Can you plan to live in an area where housing costs less than where you are now? For instance, if you sell a house in the south of England and buy one in the north you will release capital. It won't be worth it if your family and friends are all in the south. You may be able to sell your house and rent accommodation from a housing association which provides housing for the disabled. Or organise such an association.

Then there is the family life pattern to assess. If the disabled partner has to stay at home can he/she cope with the children well enough to enable the able-bodied partner to go out to work? Running a house is physically hard work and help will be needed here. Many home-bound disabled people can cope with local shopping if using an electrically-propelled wheelchair, or using a car with hand-controls. Cooking is usually possible but vacuuming, floor-washing, cleaning baths, bedmaking and changing are very difficult if not impossible.

All this should be discussed by the family group together. Include all the children. Let everyone speak. Let all ask questions. Listen to each other. *No interruptions* even if you disagree. It's most important that everyone feels that they are important members of a team. In times of stress there may well be tactless remarks but let them pass. Let all the family know in terms they can understand how and why life is about to change. 'We'll see more of Mum/Dad now she/he isn't working and that's a good thing', is a positive contribution. Children want to know. It's the unknown that is frightening. From my long experience in counselling adolescents I know that when their family has a crisis young people are very much more distressed by being kept in ignorance than they are by being told the facts. They are valued as people if they are given the chance to share some of the burden. They grow in stature if they feel they are necessary to the family group. Beware of laying too heavy a responsibility on young shoulders though. They need room and some freedom to grow up. And be prepared—initially they will fall over each other helping and eventually all will leave jobs to everyone else and argue about whose fault it was. This is natural. Treat it lightly. Don't nag, don't whine. Bang a gong to summon the troops, line them up and list the jobs. Or ring a bell to gather the household, seat the parliament round the table and point out the problems. Offer a prize such as staying up to watch a TV programme to the first person who sees and does what has been neglected. Treat problems collectively. Let every day have some family togetherness, kindliness, time to talk. Every member will suffer in some way with the victim and this must be acknowledged and accepted.

Remember how long it can take bad medical news to sink in. Never be impatient if people forget or misremember.

The Mature Adult

This is the time when many responsibilities have been shed. The mortgage has been paid off or nearly so, the children are moving on to their own path, the aged parents are in sheltered accommodation, your income belongs to you again. This is the eagerly-awaited time for which you had made so many plans. It is hard when disability threatens to turn sour the fruits of a lifetime's work just as you reach out to enjoy them. Hopefully you can plan for yourself and your partner without having to

15

consider young children and their future. If you train yourself to think and talk of this as retiring early you may well find it an interesting and enjoyable challenge. The house you now choose will probably be your last and must be well chosen. It needs to be easy to run, convenient to use, economical, near to chemist, doctor, neighbours, shops, friends and family. Possibly some part-time work using your experience may be available but it is more likely that you will feel that the rest of your life is for living, not for working. Ask friends and relatives to help you think out the things which can be done to ease your daily living. Can you turn the garden into a paved area with a border of easy-care shrubs and bulbs? Can you make a sheltered walkway from garage to house? Can you make a shed or 'chair-port' for an electric wheelchair and its charger? It's surprising how often projects like these bring in neighbourly help or advice and information about bargain supplies. Make a list of what you need, call in Social Services for advice, find out what you are entitled to, and when it's all organised settle down to living a new life, as full as you can make it.

You will find that as your contemporaries gradually become retired you merge into the landscape, become one of the crowd. They fail to foresee, are taken by surprise by, problems that you have already solved. It is surprising how many people choose to retire to, to grow old in, houses that are not easy for the old. When a car can no longer be used, the walk to the nearest bus stop becomes longer with every load of shopping. Energy to organise house selling and buying is no longer abundant. It's a poor life that is spent planning for catastrophe but as we grow older we should remember that human bodies, unlike good violins and wine, do not improve with age, and plan accordingly. We all dread dependency in old age. *Once you have mastered the technique of being disabled, you can function longer than most* and old age is not such a problem.

Generally Speaking

Whatever age you are when you become disabled there are some very helpful rules.

Regret will eat into the life, the spirit, the being of victim and of carer if you allow it to exist. Do not allow it. Be positive in your attitude, your thinking, your planning and your social approach to friends and to strangers. Stern control is needed and practice makes perfect. In hospital I met a girl who'd had polio at the age of 10 months. She was glad she'd never run as she felt she couldn't miss what she'd never known. I, disabled at 22, was glad I'd had the experience as I could recall what it felt like, could re-experience it. Is it 'better to have loved and lost than never to have loved at all'? Whatever you feel on this question don't let distant fields be greenest. There are good intelligent reasons for believing one's own garden to be the greenest of all; it gives one the strength to go on gardening.

It is no consolation, when you are struggling to get on an even keel, to be told (as so many would-be comforters insist on telling you) that... 'it would be far worse if..' or 'my friend knows someone who's got what you've got as well as...'. Learn to stop this. Try saying, 'Oh dear, I've to take my medicine in seven minutes and I've run out of the acid-drops/toffee/chocolate drops I use to help me swallow it. Would you help? Could you get me something from that corner shop?' That should get rid of the uncomforting comforter and the goodies will make a nice little surprise for your carer when he/she returns. (But beware—we disabled people should not get fat). It is tempting to let off steam by exploding at the tactless but you'll probably regret it if you do. You will acquire a reputation for being difficult and when you can't get out and about as freely as you used to do, you don't have the chance to be seen being sociable and the reputation for being difficult may stick and grow and put off people who could become good friends. It is usual to find that when you are first disabled or ill many people come to visit. It can be very exhausting but stay cheerful! The numbers who call will decrease in time and you will be left with a small number of true friends with whom you'll feel easy. When you are having a large number of visitors you and your family should practise a few polite ways of dismissing guests who have stayed too long for your ease. 'It is so kind of you to call, we've enjoyed your visit but John must rest before his relatives come tonight'. 'I've so much enjoyed your being here but the doctor said I had to sleep every afternoon at present, I'm sure you'll understand'. 'Will it seem very odd if I ask you to go so that we can change the bed? Aunt Fanny insists on doing our laundry at present and she's calling for it in an hour. She so wants to help and we love seeing her'. 'The doctor said he'd come this afternoon to give me an injection so we want to be ready, he's so busy...'. Or just nod off!

4. House and Home, Safe and Sound?

There are many trains of thought in this important area. Homes are not necessarily permanent features, especially if there are aging parents or growing and departing children to take into account. As families grow and shrink over time, housing needs (as well as income) change. Careers often involve removing when you are promoted and money is always needed for aids and care, so earning as much as possible is important. Houses are their owners' principal capital asset and must be saleable. Some people feel that too many built-in aids for disabled people repel buyers. There is so much talk of the 'special needs' of disabled people that it is casually assumed that what they need is of no use to others. But when steps were replaced with slopes so that wheelchairs could get into public places, young mothers with prams were delighted. In any house the disabled person's refuge or living area or castle can safely be advertised as a granny-flat, a bachelor pad, the teenager's den, the family's 'rumpus room', or the hobby-horse rider's 'don't let the kids in there' place. After all, if you can wheel in a disabled person you can also wheel in the potter's kiln, or granny, or the model railway supports, or the twins, or the CB radio equipment. An extra loo, washbasin or shower are blessings in any home.

If you need it, it is possible to have a stair-lift or a box-lift, or an extension to the house for a downstairs bedroom, loo, shower or bathroom. Grants are available from the local council for necessary adaptations but you must plan and seek permission first. If you begin the work without permission you forfeit your right to a grant. Too many inadequate workmen have left an expensive mess to be cleared up at the local council's expense. Social Services know who is experienced in doing this kind of work in your area. They will not object to your choosing your own firm if it is known to be reliable. Also it is possible for local councils to use bulk orders and so save money.

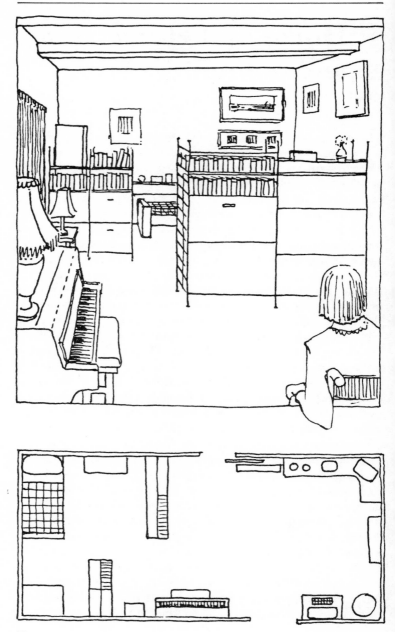

The Muscular Dystrophy Group have produced an excellent set of eight books for the disabled, one of which gives a thorough and clear account of what you are entitled to in the way of house-adaptation. It tells you how to plan and apply for permission and for a grant. Many special groups produce excellent sensible books which deserve to be more widely known. Publicity is expensive and so the books are only advertised to the groups' own members.

Be warned that the more suitable and convenient and comfortable you make your own home the more difficult it will be to leave it. Holidays can be ruined if the lift 'Oh yes, we have a lift' is too small to take your wheelchair. I have twice found that my 'en suite' bathroom, booked at an extra cost I really could not afford, was quite useless because of two steps or an extra narrow door. Train corridors, aeroplane gangways and loos are too narrow for any wheelchairs except for one designed especially by Newton for the Spastics Society. The wheelchair is light, folds up small, costs under £200 and is too narrow for me as my shoulders are broader than an aeroplane gangway! While you are young and relatively active it may be a good idea to travel more and not make home so snug and 'you-shaped' that you settle down into it too soon. When you are older, tireder, a little more affluent, use all the experience you've gathered to plan the perfect 'you-shaped' place. When the rating officer came to assess my converted sixteenth-century cottage he said it was a super bachelor pad! That was not my intention and he must have thought it was wasted on me. Here are things you need to think about.

Doors are a great nuisance. If left open they let out heat and bring in draughts. If you walk with stick, crutches or a walking-frame or if you use a wheelchair, it is very difficult to reach back to the door-handle to pull the door closed behind you. If one hand pulls the door and one hand wheels the chair, the chair goes in a circle. Sliding doors are simpler and safer for anyone and specially for the disabled. If they are 'top-hung' there's no danger of fluff from carpets getting into the slide. Furniture can be placed so that there is just room for the door to slide behind it.

Open-plan living makes movement easier. I have done away with walls and doors as I live alone. Furniture at right-angles to the main walls separates the living area from the sleeping area. The 'bookcases' on the plan are almost six feet tall, have drawers and cupboards in the lower half and books along both sides of all the shelves. Guests at parties are invited to spread around but it is interesting that most acknowledge a barrier and behave as though there were a closed door.

A co-operative builder or joiner with listening ears will grasp your needs, offer ideas, accept yours and be well worth his cost. Talk through your problems and he will make things your height, your size and when you remove he can take them to the new place and fit them for you again. Be sure to get a full costing first so that you can have it done in stages that are easy for you financially. Social Services can only help if they are consulted before you order things. They are always helpful but the money often runs out before the end of the financial year so they have problems. They are in the business of enabling you to live in your own home and will supply level access, stair-lifts, box-lifts, ground-floor plumbing, but *not* room-divider furniture!

Safe and Sound?

Homes are very dangerous places. Statistics show that most accidents happen in the home and disabled people are especially vulnerable.

Crutches, sticks and walking frames are tipped with rubber so that they are stable when in contact with the ground. If the tip catches on a mat or carpet edge you will fall as the stick stumbles. The rubber tips are going to catch on rugs, mats, long-pile carpets, carpet edges and door-sills. Get rid of all of them. There are lower, smoother door-sills for front and back doors. Strangely, this outlawing of mats and rugs was a great stumbling-block for one of my disabled friends. His wife had a flamboyant taste in decor and was fond of her rugs and mats. 'I'll move them when you're going in or out.....You can surely walk round that rug?' But the partner is not always there when the phone rings, or the doorbell. When there are people about there is not always space to circumnavigate a rug. If you are taken ill suddenly and make a bee-line for the bathroom you really can't be expected to remember mats.

A particular danger point is where one carpet meets another, for instance where lounge and hall carpets meet. A metal strip is usually put over the join and may be enough for stick or frame users. When wheelchairs turn they drag carpets and they must turn in doorways and halls. The carpet soon pulls out from the metal strip. There is a broad sticky tape made to fasten under carpet edges to stop them fraying and it's available in several colours. Put it *under* as well as *over* the carpet joins and it should hold them together, giving you a smooth ride over the join.

Wheelchairs and *carpets* do *not* get on well together. Notice when you're shopping how hard it is to wheel on carpet. Many a friend has said to me when shopping, 'Have you put the brakes on? Is something catching on the wheel?' The answer is, 'No, we're now on carpeted floor.' Carpet pile drags on the wheels and wheelchairs eat the pile from good quality carpet. Wilton or Axminster best quality will be bald within seven years. (Mine were). The easiest surfaces to wheel on are wood or linoleum or cork, but if you walk at all be careful on these surfaces. Any water or steam makes them treacherously slippery especially for stick or crutch rubbers. There is a new non-slip lino which is very good (but rather gaudy!). Even quarry tiles are dangerous when they are wet. If you must have carpets then try a bonded man-made fibre, or looped cord. The easiest to move on, but not to clean, is coconut matting.

Trailing flexes are hazardous and a high price to pay for the convenience of the gadgets they connect. They collect dust, twist round each other and are the best stick-trippers in the house. The plug socket is another problem if it's down on the skirting boards. It's the silliest place for sockets as it's a temptation to the toddler and impossible for the old or the stiff or the disabled person. Ask any electrician why they're there and the answer seems to be that they always have been. 'You don't want them halfway up the wall, do you?' The answer to that is a firm 'Yes'. If it looks unsightly, mask them with furniture until electricians get their ideas flowing and learn to put them in clusters in channels in the wall or into built-in boxes with sliding fronts. Flexes too need a rethink. Reading lamps which are moved to

23

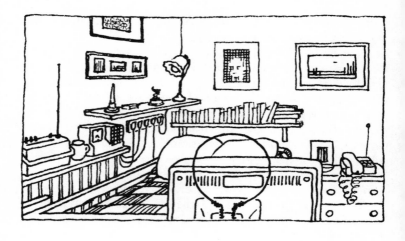

the place where you need light invariably have short flexes. TV aerial and video flexes intertwine and you may wish to have in reach as well an electric blanket, microwave oven, telephone, tea-maker, radio, record-player, alarm-clock. Unplugging and replugging knits flexes together and knocking the contents of the electric kettle over the electric blanket could be the last thing you do! A fire blanket or a small fire extinguisher should be in reach. Caravan shops have many kinds.

Pulling curtains or *blinds* isn't easy or safe. It would be if the room had no furniture but as things are you have to meander and stretch. If cords are fitted both curtains can be operated from one position. The cord can be trailed over a hook fixed to the wall some distance from the window if that is an easier position to reach.

Furniture can be arranged to help you to do short regularly-recurring house-walks without sticks or walking-frame. A bookcase against one wall will give support on one side. A settee back will give support on the other. The furniture must always be in the right place of course. If you lose your balance you grab instinctively for the usual support and come a cropper if it's out of line. If you use a wheelchair, train everyone to put on the brakes when they have moved it (if you are not in it to do it yourself).

Cushions, blankets and *knee-rugs* should be freely available so that if you fall you can pull them around yourself and be warm and comfortable until help arrives. I always have books around as well as in my bag so that I can read until someone comes. Time passes more quickly if you are interested in a book, and warm enough. It helps rescuers if you are calm and interested even though you may be in some pain.

The likeliest and literally the hardest place to fall is in the bathroom or loo. There's a cold hard floor and a shortage of cushions and rugs to pull around you. But there is an advantage to a cold hard floor—you can slither and slide on it to more public, carpeted and upholstered territory. If you can pull yourself to your feet, baths and loos are very stable objects on which to heave, press or pull. A washbasin is not. It will easily pull off the wall. It is good insurance to fit a steel or wooden support to help take the strain should it ever be necessary.

The kitchen is a problem place which needs more planning than anywhere else. It is the most dangerous room in the house. Planning for it is referred to in 'Where do you need help?' (Chap. 5). If you are disabled and working in the kitchen it is much easier to work using an electrically-propelled wheelchair. One hand controls the chair, leaving the other hand free to hold milk jug or pan or kettle. Self-propelled chairs need two hands to move them so there is danger if the turkey spits fat as it's taken from the oven and carrying milk is a splashy business. If a boiling kettle splutters people step back. The wheelchair-user needs two hands to take off the brakes (which should be on when lifting boiling kettles or pans) before using the hands to propel the chair back. For this reason I disagree with most books of design I've read which aim to get the wheelchair-user's feet under the working-surface. All spills obey gravity and the gravy lands in your lap. Scalded thighs are the last thing you need. Sideways on is safer and you can move along more easily—in fact you only need to go forward and backward, not back and turn and forward and backward. Have a tray on your lap for some things. There are trays which fit on to wheelchairs but they restrict your vision and increase the likelihood of your footrests carving up doorframes and furniture.

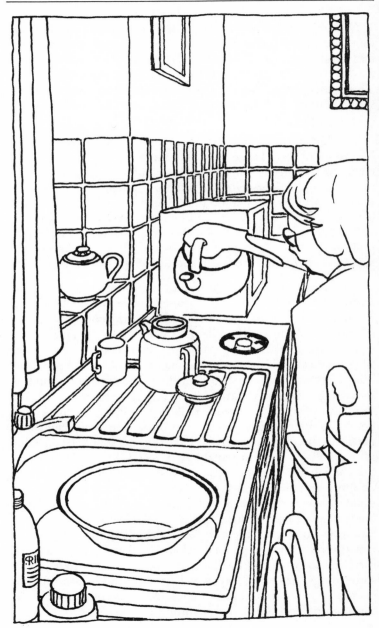

Getting into the haven. Assuming that you've got rid of steps and have slopes into your home there are still a few hazards to consider. Weather throws up many problems. Ice, snow, driving rain and gusting winds all destroy balance. Make as much shelter as you can afford between the garage door and the house door. Consider a wall, a half-wall, fencing, a trellis with shrubs growing behind it, a roofed walkway. Never plan until you know the direction of the prevailing wind. Remember that in built-up areas the north-east wind does not necessarily attack you from the geographical north-east. Local hills as well as buildings tunnel winds. It's wise but not always possible to live in a house for a year before spending money on strong protection against the worst weather. A hazard I've never conquered is the green deposit that collects on garden paths. Doing without growing things is one unpalatable solution.

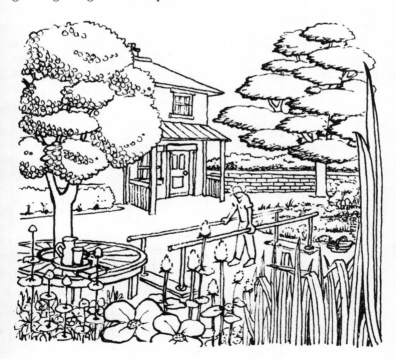

5. Where Do You Need Help?

There is an incredibly large body of inventions to help disabled people in the home and out of it. In the Appendix there are addresses of places where you may see aids on display and where you may write to get booklets and catalogues. In this chapter I hope to set you thinking.

The Loo

The place we most long to visit alone! There is a vast collection of rails—they even come in glorious technicolour to match your plumbing or wallpaper. A rail at each side of the loo may be enough if fixed at the angle which suits you. There are rails

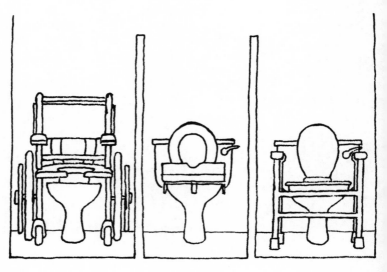

which screw to the wall behind the throne and they can be pulled down for use and slotted upright again out of other people's way. There are sets of rails which can be fixed round the toilet and some of them are designed to be easily unscrewed so you can take them on holiday or when visiting friends.

For those who find modern loo-seats far too low, there are sets of rails with a loo-seat attached which fit round and over the low seat. These are available with rubber feet or with castors. Another solution to the problem is a deep plastic loo-seat which fits into and clips on to the pot, replacing the seat at a higher level. It is light to carry but very bulky. Other people can perch on it too, or can remove it and then (hopefully!) replace it.

There are shower-chairs made from a loo-seat on four legs and a short-legged version which can be used in the bath. There is a splendid wheelchair made to be used in the shower as well as over the loo and it is a self-propelled chair. We have provided pictures of many aids because a handyman may prefer to produce his/her own version of the ideas with special refinements to suit individual needs.

If you meet a public loo with no facilities for disabled people try this. Put your feet either side of the footrests and then turn up the footrests. Wheel forward until the front of the wheelchair seat is touching the front of the loo-seat. (The footrests will go either side of the pot). Then shuffle forward on to the throne, as though leaping on to horseback over the horse's tail. It isn't comfy but it works when you're desperate. It's safe as you're fenced in by the loo-tank in front and the wheelchair armrests beside you and the wheelchair back behind you. If the loo-door opens inwards you have to leave it open but people in Britain are good at looking the other way or even at melting away until you are out again.

I've been disabled around Britain for almost 40 years and am happy to be independent in lavatories, which is as well because I've never been offered help, though no doubt it would have been given if I'd asked for it. I've visited Canada twice for five weeks in all and every time I wheeled into a 'comfort station' I was offered help. 'I'll be happy to give you any assistance you might require' was always said by some member of the public. And all public places had wheelchair loos. In the Toronto Art Gallery I was festooned with shopping and wheeled into the 'disabled' loo, both to use it and to reorganise the shopping. Almost at once there was a rat-tat-tat on the door and a cheerful voice called 'Lady in there? Lady in there? Do you need any help? I'll gladly assist if you need me to. Are you O.K.?' I also had shop doors held open for me there however rushed people were. They held a door and sped on their way—you can't rely on that happening in this country.

The Bath

Baths are treacherous. They are slippery to begin with and wetness and soap make bad worse. Bath salts, bath cubes and bubble-bath are disastrously skid-causing. Whatever you hold on to will be slippery if your hands are wet. A steam extractor fan helps to reduce the bathroom's moisture content but makes it feel a little chilly.

Flooring. Carpet gets soggy and isn't easy for wheelchairs to turn on. Quarry tiles are good but cold if bare feet touch them, and you can't risk bath mats. The new non-slip lino is very good. Cork tiles are excellent, being warmer to the touch than most floor coverings. I was very pleased with my cork tiles until I found their major disadvantage. Woodworm can have a beanfeast underneath and you are unaware of them until a guest's foot goes through the floor!

Bath mats which attach to the base of the bath by means of suckers are the cheapest form of anti-skid device. But they are hard to clean and they get gungy. Then the suckers, while still clinging to the bath-base, slither and skid. So always have a new one ready. There are strips and flower shapes which you can stick on to the bath and these last for several years before wearing off. In an emergency put a towel in the bottom of the bath to reduce skid.

Rails come in a variety of sizes and shapes, some being made to fit across the bath.

A *board* fitted between the wall and the round end of the bath is useful to slide up on to (or down into the bath from). If you don't use a wheelchair have a strong wooden chair with arms to flop on to when you're safely out of the bath. You need a safe perch when drying yourself and getting your breath back.

Stools or *shelves* which lodge halfway in the bath exist in many forms, some of which we've illustrated. You can use them as a halfway house getting in and getting out, or sit on them while you bath. If you wish to wallow in the water, to soak and wriggle and move as you can move in water, which removes the effects of gravity and makes limbs lighter, then you need strong arms to heave out the perch when you're in the bath and heave it back in when you wish to get out. Putting an ordinary wooden stool in the bath to sit on is *not* a good idea. When you try to sit on it to get out, the stool floats! And if you let out all the water then you miss the support it gives you as you heave yourself up. Always leave the bath water in the bath—it gives helpful support and is softer to fall on to than the empty bath would be. It does make a wet mess on walls and floor if you flop back in to it but it gives you fewer bruises.

If you use a stool (the purpose-built kind) or a shelf which lodges against the sides of the bath, make certain that your bath will withstand the pressure. Plastic baths won't. Choose a new bath at your leisure before buying the gadgets rather than have a catastrophe dictate a new bath in a hurry. One city council built old people's bungalows and put in plastic baths that wouldn't take the strain imposed by bath-seats. The solution? They removed the baths and hired buses to take the old people to public baths! (There are no prizes for thinking up better solutions).

Hoists can be attendant-operated or self-operated. Some have sets of slings for arms, legs and torso and appear daunting. Some use inflatable cushions which work electrically, deflating to get you in and reflating to lift you out. Mecanaid of Gloucester fix a support to the floor on which swings a chair which moves up and down as you turn a knob. This is illustrated on page 32. Mangar Aids of Presteigne, Powys, make a portable bath-lift which requires no fixtures and no fitting. It can be operated by the disabled person alone or by a carer.

The Chiltern Mini-Bathroom (Chiltern House, Wedgwood Road, Bicester) is incredibly compact. The unit can be installed in the corner of a bedroom or utility room or bathroom. There is

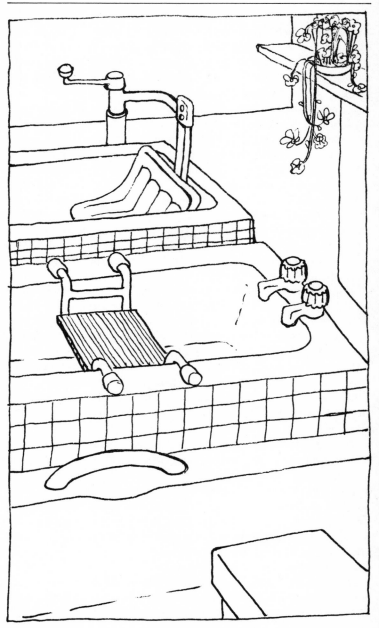

a lavatory over which the wheeled shower-chair will park. There is a pull-down washbasin and an overhead shower. All this is housed in a cabinet which has sealed half-doors and a shower curtain. Safety measures include thermostatic water temperature control, a pump to remove waste water, and an antiflood device

Alarm system. However primitive it is, do have one. A whistle to blow, a dinner-gong to bang, a bell to ring. I used to sit in the bath after bathing to shampoo my hair using a shower-hose which fixed on to both taps. One evening the shower-hose plopped off the hot tap and I suffered a severe scalding of my left foot. My yells went for nothing as my parents were watching the 'Last Night of the Proms' on TV and I was outsung by the massed promenaders.

The Bed

This is the friendly haven which is easier to get on and off than anything else you occupy, because it's soft to land on and big enough to roll on to. It is good if there is enough space underneath it for wheelchair footrests and feet during

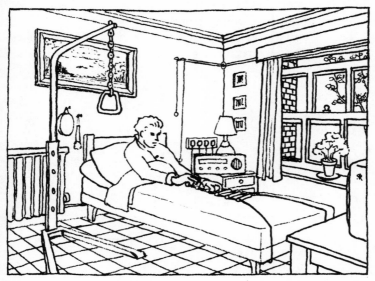

bedmaking. Divans lack this and are very cumbersome to move. Beds with castors are easy to move and lethal to move on to unless placed into a corner where two sides are against walls. If the bed is lower than the wheelchair seat put a board under the mattress to raise it, or put a wooden block with a hollow under each leg of the bed.

Rails are made to fit on to bedsides to stop people falling out and they are a great help when you are turning over in bed, too. It's easier to pull on a rail than it is to pull on the mattress. If you buy bunk beds you can have one in a guest bedroom and use the upper bed (on the floor of course!) yourself. Its built-in rail helps you turn over and either end of the bed can be used as the top end, so the rail can be whichever side you choose.

Practise rolling on and off your bed when someone is there. Don't let them help but have them there during the practice as a form of insurance. Experiment until you find a safe way of transferring alone. Find ways of doing all you can when someone else is there and you will have the confidence to do it alone. If parents or carers are too protective they can unwittingly encourage risk-taking in their absence. We all treasure our independence, however limited it is. I speak from experience in this. Don't take risks when you are alone—it gives your guardian angel too much exercise!

To pull yourself up in bed use a rope-ladder or try a 'monkey-pole' (See the picture on page 33). The balkan beam has a

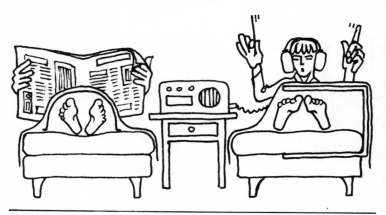

multitude of uses, as can be seen in any orthopaedic ward, as well as being useful to pull you up in bed.

There are many variously-shaped pillows to support backs, as well as fleeces of specially-made fibres to prevent sore skin. Duvets are light but you can use frames to keep bedding off your toes and legs.

Dressing and Undressing

Wear clothes of strong colour made of good material to cheer yourself up. Snap up sales remnants and get a collection of easy-to-sew economical patterns. Find a dressmaker or learn to be one. Handsewing may be easier than machining. Use easy zips with large tabs and good-sized buttons and buttonholes if your hands are stiff. Wrap-round skirts are easy to put on and take off. Jogging suits are designed to be easy to pull on and off and are now available in velour and velvet so they're attractive enough for parties. All 'leisure wear' is easy to wear. Try kaftans, tabards, housecoats, fisherman's smock, crew-neck or boatneck sweaters in fine wool or silk. Collect large or long silk scarves and fluffy shawls because they are the easiest way to adjust to changing temperatures. Swish trousers can elegantly cover inelegant but warm long johns, legwarmers, wool stockings, handknitted socks as well as high boots. Loose velvet jackets look attractive and can cover the warm wool jumper. You will be chilly at parties because you can't move around and find warm places! Batwing sleeves are easy to wear as you can get your elbow out first. Trousers with no zip but elastic at the waist are easier to deal with.

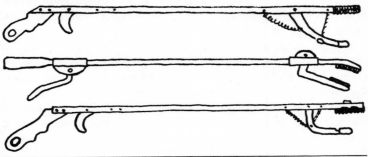

Don't choose lace-up shoes if you can't get down there; use velcro straps instead and fasten them with a 'helping hand' or 'easireach' (see picture on page 35). Buckles and zips are easier than laces. If you hand-propel a wheelchair sailing gloves are great. The palms have reinforced leather, the backs are net and there are no finger-ends so you can show your nail varnish and stop your hands getting corny. Pockets are invaluable and lots of pockets means no need for a hand-bag which is often awkward when there is a struggle with steps or in and out of cars and wheelchairs.

The Kitchen

Whether or not you have your kitchen designed round your wheelchair (or your need to sit down to work) depends on who's in charge of kitchen work and who helps. If you're in charge and the kitchen is designed round you, don't opt out and leave your partner to cope too often. If the working-surfaces, cooker and sink are too high for comfort the cheapest solution is to put a firm, deep upholstery cushion on to your wheelchair seat. If washer, fridge and freezer are too low mount them on wooden blocks. They don't, in my experience, sit too safely on the mass-produced runners which are advertised a lot. If cupboards are too high they can be lowered. Or store on the work-surface the things you most often use and put on the shelves things rarely used. You can ask people to get them down for you when, say, the jam-making season, or Christmas, arrives. The 'helping hand' can be frustrating in the kitchen as it's awkward to manage a weighty glass jar at the far end of the 'helping hand' and, perhaps for this reason, the grip is not quite wide enough for many kitchen items like coffee jars.

If surfaces are raised, other people can still use them easily; if things are lowered other people have problems. Give helpers a chair to sit on and they'll manage. If they say 'Oh, I can't wash up sitting down!' the answer is they must, you have to, anything's possible, have a new experience! There is a set of kitchen units and sink which can be raised and lowered but it needs a spanner, screwdriver and considerable time; it's not to be done daily.

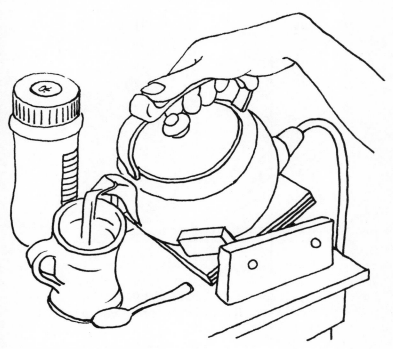

Kitchen gadgets

We all know how one woman's favourite gadget is left to moulder at the back of another woman's cupboard, unused. The golden rule is—TRY IT BEFORE YOU BUY IT. Food processors, slow cookers, mixers, liquidisers and deep fryers are expensive to buy, bulky to store, heavy to pull towards you and uncomfortably high to reach to put things into them (when you're sitting). You may well need a specially low surface for these. Borrow one and try it before you buy one. I've always found that the cheap, lightweight, hand-held gadgets are easiest to use, wash and store accessibly. Depending on one's particular difficulty there are one-handed tin-openers (mine is the best I've ever used of any kind), large-handled cutlery, electric knives, non-slip mats, prongs to transfix slippery eatables while carving them up, tilting platforms for kettles and teapots (see the picture this page), wire pastry-blenders which rub fat into flour for

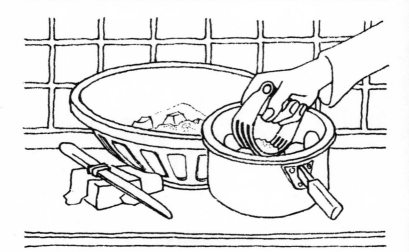

scones as well as mashing potatoes (see picture above), and things to get tops off jars and bottles. Occupational therapists can show you catalogues of all these and more. Or write to the addresses in the Appendix or put your problem to a handyman or invent things yourself.

The *microwave oven* is worth investigating for the physically handicapped. It's portable and can be used wherever you have a 13-amp plug and a table. Try it in the bedroom or dining room or kitchen. There's no door-handle, just press a switch. If you see the milk begin to boil up, press a switch and it subsides at once. You can cook on the dish you eat from, make coffee in the cup you drink it from, so there's much less washing up. A plateful of food warms through in a minute or two, remaining moist and tasty. Small quantities are cooked very quickly indeed. The method of cooking needs study, and men take to it with enthusiasm often because they don't have to unlearn or rethink as most women do. There are lots of classes and demonstrations at present.

Transporting Things

It's dull to eat in the kitchen and more fun in a sunny window with a view of the neighbourhood or near the TV, especially if there's any snooker or cricket. Get a trolley—not, needless to say, the wilful supermarket variety! Some have a high rail you can hold while walking. It needs large reliable wheels which will take carpet edges in their stride (if you have any carpet edges) without spilling the milk. Tie to it a rubber ring (the kind you buy at pet shops to throw for your dog) and put the ring under one of the wheels when you arrive at your destination so you can stabilise the trolley. You can use the trolley for food, phone, hobbies, books, painting materials, binoculars.

If you use a walking-frame attach two or three bags to it. Bags made of patchwork and lined with patchwork are strong, long-lasting and washable. Bag handles can be tied to the frame or held to it with crocodile-clips which cost a few pence each at DIY stores or garages. If you use a wheelchair, hang a bag from each handle with a short tie so that the bag doesn't rub on the wheels (this wears a hole on the bag and acts as a brake on the chair needless to say). You can also have a bag with its two handles hanging on the wheelchair's two handles so that the bag goes right across the back of the chair. Swivelling round to put things in and get them out is good exercise for the waistline. Thus equipped you can carry knitting, newspaper and nosh without mixing them up in transit. If you walk with sticks sling a long-handled bag across each shoulder—but don't rest one on each shoulder or they flop off and give you a balancing problem. It is

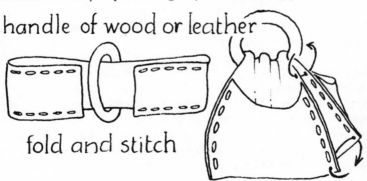

handle of wood or leather

fold and stitch

stitch at top and at bottom corners

better to put your head through the handle and then let the handle drop on to your shoulder.

Bags made from left-over furnishing fabrics are lighter than leather bags and longer lasting than plastic materials and can be stuffed full of contents. Once people know you can use fabrics you'll be well supplied—people enjoy keeping you busy and clearing out their spare rooms. On page 39 there is a plan to help you make a useful double-bag. If you can't cope hand it to Aunt Fanny and see what she makes of it.

Easy Food

Have fresh fruit nearby to quench thirst and stave off hunger and give nutrition. Cleaned, raw, grated or chopped vegetables are filling, not fattening, are fashionably fibre-full and will keep several days in polythene bags, preferably in a fridge. Red and green peppers, sprouts, cabbage, cauliflower florets and carrots are ideal for this. Tomatoes to bite can be refreshing but watch out for spurting pips and have kitchen roll ready to mop up spills before they coagulate. The tomato skin is excellent fibre so eat up! Cheese, a hard-boiled egg kept in its shell to keep it fresh until you're ready to eat it, a few plain biscuits or crackers will provide a light meal so you won't be wilting and ravenous when your carer gets in from a hard day's work.

Sweet biscuits and cake are fun but you mustn't get fat. Chocolate will rot your teeth, make your bowels sluggish, spoil your complexion, thicken your waistline as well as killing your teeth. I'm an expert on diets as I've been losing the battle of the bulge for over 30 years. You owe it to carers, if you have carers, not to get fat and heavy. It's easier to move about with difficulty if you are slim rather than stout, but if you are tall with long useless legs you have problems in moving which are not solved by being thin. A thermos of boiling water can be used on tea or packet soup or Bovril. A thermos of boiling milk can be poured on cocoa or coffee or Reddibrek or muesli. In winter a wide-necked thermos full of hot vegetable soup or porridge or rice pudding will be good central heating at mid-day. Wholemeal sandwiches can hold marmite, sardines or pilchards, cheese grated with apple, apple grated with finely-chopped dates, carrot grated with raisins, sliced meat with pickle or coleslaw, pâté if it's spread meanly. Wrap them in cling-film to keep them fresh.

Communicating

British Telecom have produced a glossy booklet on their aids for the handicapped. If you have problems with seeing, hearing or with trembling fingers they have aids you can use. Check the cost, because they can be expensive. It seems sensible to have a radio-phone in your car so you can call for help without troubling passers-by if you break down. I read about these in the booklet and rang the freephone number to make enquiries for myself as well as for you! The cost, I was told, was between three and four thousand pounds for installation as tuning was difficult and the calls cost 27 pence per unit. I gasped and said I couldn't possibly afford that and was told Social Security would pay. I can assure you that they won't and laughter rang round County Hall when I asked if anyone had asked for this facility at this price. It would take four years' of your mobility allowance to pay for it so you wouldn't have a car to put it in by then. I'm *not* arguing that it should be supplied but question the wisdom and sense of printing this as a useful service to the disabled. If the cost were printed first it would be fairer as you wouldn't read on. I've broken down and been repaired at the roadside for years and can go on doing so. Citizens' Band Radio is an interesting possible alternative.

Remember how easy it is to use the phone when you're in all day. Follow business rules, no calls at all until after one o'clock. Phone bills are a dreaded thud on the door mat.

There are many alarm systems being developed so that you can call for help if you live alone and fall or become ill. Until recently you had to fall or become ill near your phone. Now there are transistor-links to computers and telephone exchanges and wardens which are being tried out in sheltered accommodation and in neighbourhood schemes. You can wear an alarm-call which is no larger than a piece of jewellery. There are also battery-operated alarm-calls which give tongue on your behalf when you need help. It's wise to let your neighbours hear it so they'll recognise it as an SOS. Ask around before you spend. Ask Social Services if you can be a guinea-pig in any experiments that are going forward in your area.

The bathroom and loo are likely places to fall so I had a telephone jack-plug placed there. Three or four nights were disturbed by a wailing noise. I don't believe in ghosts but my small dog did and she howled in horror. When my new phone developed a fault I asked the engineer to investigate the bathroom jack-plug and he found condensation on the line inside the wall behind the tiles. (In the film *The Women* made in 1938 one character spends much of her time in the bath on the phone. In England in the mid-1980s she wouldn't have been able to do so!) My phone link was built in during the renovation of an old cottage. I now have the jack-plug outside the bathroom door and the phone wire trails across the floor, adding to the likelihood of my coming a cropper. I'm *now* told that the answer is a cordless phone but they cost over £100 and as it wasn't suggested when I was planning and spending money I can't afford it. This is a long-winded way of saying that *you must pursue what you need with tenacity*. No one will think *for* you. You must see the snags. British Telecom will not. They will expect you to spend until you have what you need.

Communicating micro-technology, chips with everything

This is a rapid growth area and you need expert advice to be sure you know what you need. This is the world of software, hardware, graphics, floppy discs, word processing, speech synthesisers, daisy wheels and so on. It's a young world, a fun world and a coming world. Chips are small, cheap, adaptable and can help you control machines which can do what you can't. You may be enabled to write, turn pages, operate a wheelchair, use TV, turn lights on and off, draw curtains or answer a door. Machines will speak if you can't see, produce written words if you can't hear and print copies of their writing and drawing if you need them.

Control can be exercised by a finger, a toe, a mouth-held

pointer, head movement to left or right, eye movement, blowing or sucking. Some machines will respond to a particular voice. It's clear, therefore, that each machine is tailor-made to fit particular needs and abilities and you may need training in order to use a machine effectively. All this sounds complicated but many aids are light and portable so you can travel with the small aid while using the larger, more versatile model at home.

Synthesised voices have been difficult to understand but they are being improved all the time so don't 'write them off' if you've met a poor one. Print can be converted to Braille and there are machines which read books aloud. Word processors print on a screen words which then are typed, corrections can be made and then the final copy can be printed. They even check the spelling.

Machines will teach you, play games with you. You can gain access to BBC's Ceefax and ITV's Oracle through a machine which converts the text to Braille. You can make phone calls through the RNID telephone exchange. This computer world is

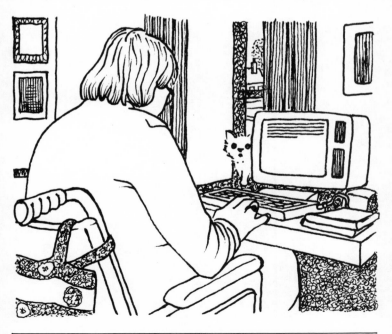

a vast area of opportunity for achieving things yourself and is a highway to job opportunity, in accountancy for example, if you become highly skilled. Many of the systems have been developed by disabled people who needed them and who now supply them to others.

So discuss this area of help with your doctor, your physiotherapist, experts in electronics from university or colleges of further and higher education. Find out what is available that might help you. Dr Hugh Grenfell has used computers to stimulate paralysed muscles and some wheelchair-users can sometimes walk a few steps with the aid of micro-technology. Development goes on all the time. There's no VAT to pay on things which are designed for disabled people to use because of their disability.

Don't dream about it, find out about it.

6. Getting Out and About and Rescued

Getting out is a very valuable and important activity. The small change of human intercourse is important. Not every human contact should be a deep, meaningful or positive relationship. It does the mind good to rub against very differing attitudes from those usually encountered. Find out how people feel and think who don't feel and think as you do and you will have more to think about when you are alone. Getting out and about gives life interest, a little danger perhaps and the possibility of a host of new activities. Before you consider the many tempting types of transport think about *where* you're going and *why*.

The Self-propelled Wheelchair

This is supplied by the DHSS to all who need one. It is possible to buy them but on the whole they are very alike. You may be advised to propel yourself so that you exercise and keep strong arms and chest. Now that sport for disabled people is blossoming there is some rethink in design. It is high time! The self-propelled wheelchair is loaded with prongs and knobs on which laundry catches as you fold it, clothes catch as you shuffle on and off it, bags catch as you load and unload it. The backrest leaves your back without support just where it most needs it. The seat is iron-hard and curves down in the middle. The brakes, one on each wheel, are primitive—five sets of nuts and bolts on each operate a flat piece of metal. The tyres need pumping up, although you can get flexible inserts to avoid this hard labour. The footrests come off when they're turned up for you to stand or sit and they test the patience of the steadiest character when being persuaded back on. The footrests jam when you fold the chair unless you remember to fold them up first (this is when they like to shoot off

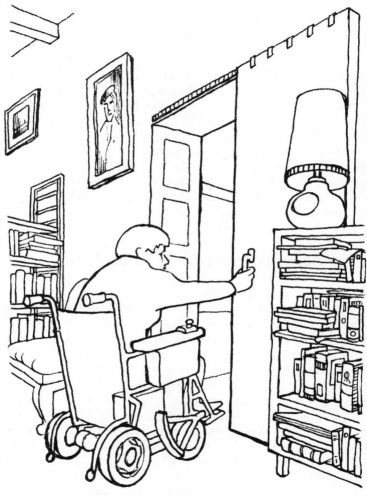

A middle-price-range electrically-propelled chair.

the chair). Footrests have sharp edges at the front, side and corner which carve grooves in walls and furniture and doors and doorways because you can't see the edges of the footrests as you propel the chair especially if you have anything on your lap such as laundry, shopping or the useful trays which fit over the armrests.

The usual folding is side up to side but you must seize the centre front and centre back of the seat to persuade the chair to fold. When opening it again the side of the seat must be pressed, *not* the armrests, though you can't easily get at the seat-sides as the armrests are in the way. If you add a little comfort such as a cushion, sheepskin or back-support, all this has to be removed before you can fold and transfer the chair to a car. Disabled young people can get from the DHSS a beautiful low-backed, low-arm, light, bright red sports wheelchair—*if* they are involved in sports.

If you are advised to use a self-propelling chair and don't like the DHSS provision, shop around a long time before you buy. The Spastic Society has had a chair designed which is narrow enough to go through train and plane doors and corridors. The large wheels can be pulled off, leaving the chair narrower, running on four small wheels, and it can be pushed through narrow spaces. If, like me, you are broad in build, the chair is painfully narrow, but it does enable you to go where you couldn't go without it. It costs just under £200.

An Electrically-propelled Chair

One of these, from the middle-price range, will be a blessing in the house. You can carry the milk in one hand and steer the chair with the other. Your arms can save their energy for the housework, though one day's domestic labour will empty the batteries. It will see you to the local shops or to and round a small town in fairly level territory. A more expensive, heavy duty electrically-propelled chair will go to town, through a park, bounce up five inch high steps and do up to 30 miles on a battery charge. But it will be too bulky, too big and insufficiently manoeuvrable to use in the average house. All types of electrically-propelled scooters and chairs are suitable for meeting rooms, clubs, pubs and libraries.

Petrol-driven Three-wheelers

These are strong, sturdy, noisy, vibrating and so are out of place in shops, libraries and evening classes. But they are first class for

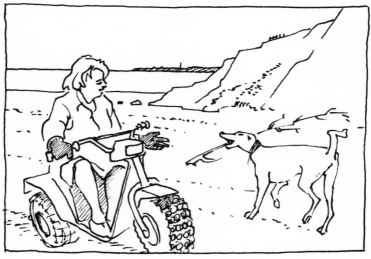

Dog-walking with a Range-Rider.

dog-walking, fresh air pursuits, football matches, cricket matches, moors and parks, and for shopping if you walk a little.

Folding wheelchairs, the electric scooters and smaller electrically-propelled wheelchairs will go into most car boots. The heavy duty electric chairs and petrol-driven three-wheelers will not. You can use a small trailer attached to the car for these if you wish to take one on holiday.

These vehicles can be purchased with your mobility allowance if you qualify for one. If you run a car as well they are an extra expense and it's up to you what you need. What enhances your quality of life most? Running the vehicles is not costly but renewing them is. They do not have a long life if you make good use of them. The batteries in a wheelchair have six months warranty and cost over £100 to renew. While you are working it is affordable but when you retire capital is soon eaten away. When retired you have more time to enjoy the freedom these vehicles give and you are likely to wear them out more quickly!

A Car

A car is comfortable and as it has extra seating you can have company—of your own choosing as it's your car! Hand controls are available but do shop around for them. Some firms keep your car for weeks (some for as long as 10 weeks) queuing for their attention and not under cover. They will not ring you when they're ready to work on it, nor agree to do it while you wait for the car. There is one firm which employs local mechanics (often disabled workers) who put on the hand controls in your own garage or in the garage where you bought the car. This is ideal and the hand controls are good, unfussy and easy to use. We give Bekker's address in the Appendix. Any make of car can be done.

Someone else has to lift your chair in and out of the car for you. Have you a helper whose back and/or heart can stand the strain? Regularly? It is wise to get hoists or mechanical aids before the strain begins to tell.

Access

Another important consideration is how many steps will you meet in your area? *Two steps = one full stop.* A strong vehicle will bounce up one step but it can't cope with more than one without a ramp. Guildford Cathedral has a ramp near every set of steps but most public buildings don't, and on the whole churches and chapels are the worst offenders in this. If you want to discover if there is a level entrance to any place ask the caretaker or the porter. He takes delivery of furniture and heavy goods and he knows exactly where you can go on the level. I challenged one architect when I had laboured long and hard to get round the school he'd designed with steps at every corner and in every corridor. His reply was that steps added visual interest. If ever he has to use a wheelchair I'm sure he will have much more visual interest than he can appreciate. Try this test. Ask your friends to tell you how many steps there are to their dentist, doctor's surgery, library, nearest cinema, public house. Then count the steps. If your results match mine, the average guess is *half* the number of steps there actually are. I think most people go up steps two at a time and count accordingly.

If you go out once a day in your chair you will extend the number of your acquaintances surprisingly. Dogs make many friends for their owners as people often talk to the dog and so give the owners the chance to join in the conversation. People become used to seeing you and comment on the weather or ask about your chair. Often they have a friend or relative who could use one and would like to know about its price, performance and maintenance. If you don't want to talk, smile and move on but if you do chat you will make innumerable links into the network of your community. If you call for your newspaper each day instead of having it delivered you will be nudged into going out each day and the change of scene and air is good for you physiologically and psychologically. If you go to a pub for a pub lunch (usually they are good value for money) you save yourself from cooking at home. You meet a variety of people, can air your views and settle the fate of the nation or listen as others put the world to rights.

Buying a Wheelchair

Before you plunge into a purchase write for every available brochure and price-list. The *Radio Times* is a prime source of advertisements and so is the monthly magazine *Handicapped Living*. Most firms offer free demonstration. Be careful though. I had a demonstration of a splendid but costly chair and the price was not revealed, in spite of my requesting it, until the demonstration. I hadn't enough money to buy it as it was much costlier than I'd guessed. Six months later I'd saved enough money and I ordered the chair. After it was delivered I was charged £38 for the 'free' delivery as I'd had a free demonstration. All firms are not as bad as this. They lost out as I did not buy from that manufacturer again but that is no help while you are caught in their system.

There are many firms in this business now and competition is keen. Beware of their habit of criticising each other's products—it is unpleasant and unhelpful. The only way to compare two or three different makes of chair is to see them at the same time and try them. If a firm of distributors sells several kinds of chair you will still find it hard to see all you wish to try. Firms do not keep a big stock and will praise the kind they have in at the time. I was told by one firm that a vehicle I wanted to try before buying had gone out of production as it had not sold well, only to find six months later that it was selling very well indeed and expanding its hold on the market except in one firm's area! Many different makes of chair use the same make of engine and control box. These are transistorised and sealed and go back to the engine maker, not the chair maker, for repair. I've never been offered a reconditioned box or engine and whether they recycle them it is not possible to say. The local firm fixes a new one. I had two control boxes for one chair I used. One was in use and one in the post! At over £200 for each box and over £3 for postage it was worth it to avoid being confined to the house for two weeks every time it went wrong. It is hard to be deprived of your freedom when you've found it again. In the Appendix there are addresses of the few places where you can try many kinds of chairs. It's worth arranging a visit but do check first that they have in stock what you want to see.

My experience of five different firms leads me to say very positively that in most cases salesmanship is better developed than after-care service. Promises are made when you buy but if you need several visits while still under guarantee, your call for help is not always well received. 'I'm not coming there twice in a fortnight' (It shouldn't go wrong twice in a fortnight). 'Whatever are you doing with it? Most people don't ring up twice in a short time like this' (I've obeyed all the instructions). 'I'll have to wait for a delivery of parts anyway so I can't come for 10 days at least'. You've no alternative but to stay at home or use taxis. At least if the chair was bought from the maker or his distributor it is under guarantee. Often one can buy vehicles at a bargain price second-hand, but there is no guarantee that they will be in good order. If you buy second-hand from a dealer he will give you a guarantee but you naturally pay more for this.

Questions to ask before buying either a new or second-hand wheelchair

Where is the nearest repair place?
How much is the call-out charge? (this ranges from £8 to £80)
How long is it between the call and your arrival?
How long is the vehicle guaranteed?
How long do they usually last?
How much are new batteries, new control box, new engines and when will I be likely to need any?
How much is insurance and what *exactly* does it cover?

The answers are not, of course, binding but they give you some idea of how hard you must save up for the next expense. The first repair my very expensive strong chair needed was after my first trip across a field. I punctured both back wheels and I requested a repair. I agreed to pay a call-out charge of £80 and said I needed two new tyres and two new inner-tubes as I'd had to ride home after the disaster. The repairman came with only one tyre and one inner-tube. I had to wait five days for the others to be delivered through the post and get a local mechanic to fit them (with great difficulty as the rear wheels are small and awkward). My bill from the firm was for £198 and the insurance only paid £28. I questioned everyone concerned by phone and post but felt I had to pay as there was no one but the maker/supplier who could do repairs of the motor and control box and I needed them to come as soon as possible when I broke down again. Without the chair I couldn't go to the shops or get fresh air or walk the dogs or meet people.

I write this to warn you that no one is in business for your benefit or for your convenience and you must accept this. Don't waste emotion on sharp business practice. You vote with your money the next time you buy and you pass on your experiences when someone asks your advice. That is all you can do. Local garages can be very helpful with repairs. If *you* order the spare parts they will usually fit them efficiently and cheaply. I have had new batteries of the correct kind ordered and fitted for *less than half* the price some chair manufacturers ask. But with the control boxes and engines you have no alternative to the manufacturer.

The vehicles are so enabling and horizon-stretching that one is woeful when they won't go.

The batteries need charging regularly and topping up with distilled water about every fortnight. They are usually under the seat so you have to prowl round your electric chair in your other wheelchair and this needs a lot of space. You may find a helpful friend or neighbour to do this for you.

Vehicles Costing Under £1000

These little scooters and runabouts are pedestrians. They are leg substitutes. There is no road tax to pay and no driving test to pass. Their speed limit is four miles an hour and they are legally entitled to go on the road only when the pavement is too narrow or too crowded or is being dug up. They are powered by two small batteries and a trickle-charger is provided. The wheels are

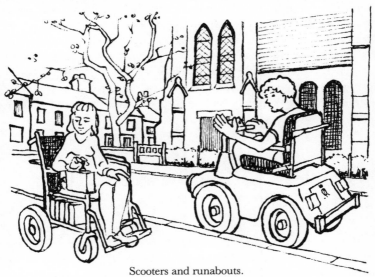

Scooters and runabouts.

small, usually with solid tyres and will climb a two or three inch high kerb (if you can find one so low!). I had some success with a plank of wood two inches thick which I laid in the gutter before I tried to get up a kerb more than a couple of inches high. I'd attached thick rope to one end of it so I could retrieve it after I'd

53

got up the step. Sometimes you 'bottom' doing this and have to be pushed on to your wheels again. The seat is a light chair with two arm-rests and it swivels to three positions so you can get on it at the easiest point for you. There's a platform for your feet, a wire basket for shopping, a clip for a walking stick. There is one reverse speed, two forward speeds but the maximum is the legal limit for pavements, four miles an hour.

The *range per battery-charge* is usually eight to twelve miles depending on your weight and how bumpy the roads are. Manufacturers test on a smooth level surface using a slender rider. If you run out of electricity you can easily disconnect the little motor and be pushed home. Often resting it for 10 minutes or so will restore a little life to get you the last few hundred yards. There is no weather-proofing—you must weather-proof yourself.

All these lightweight vehicles can be separated into smaller components and packed easily into the boot of even small cars. Batteries, seat, steering bar and platform are not too heavy to manage, separately. These vehicles are nippy, neat, useful, genteel, well-behaved indoors, look gay and young, are good in shops and the family can walk with you. They will *not* go on rough or gravelly ground, on snow or ice, or on grass, although they go nicely on bowling greens if you can find one they will let you ride on.

Vehicles Costing Between £1000 and £2000

These are the four-wheel electrically-propelled chairs, designed to be dismembered and put into a car boot. The four wheels are small. There is a kerb-climber, (one centrally or two, one at each side) which connects with the kerb and guides the chair up a five inch step.

They are compact, turn in a small space and manoeuvre well in the house. A small joy-stick steers the chair backwards, forwards and round, and this can be fitted so an attendant works

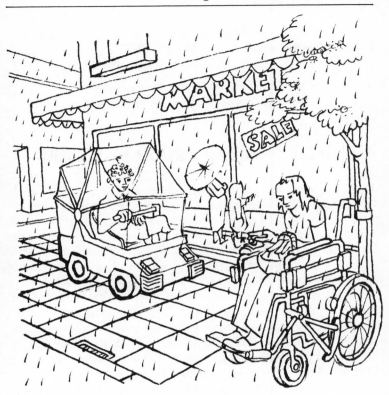

Four-wheel electrically-propelled chairs.

it if that is necessary. The battery-charger will take a few hours to charge the batteries fully and this gives approximately 14 to 16 miles (depending on your weight and the terrain covered) when the batteries are new. As they age the power diminishes. They are specially designed to be used until empty of electricity and then to be trickle-charged and so they are expensive to replace. Unless you ask for solid tyres when you order you may get the kind you have to pump up and this is exhausting. The solid tyres are blessedly puncture-proof and the air-eating tyres are not.

These chairs will *not be safe* on *rough* ground. There is usually a safety-belt although I did not get one with mine. Being used to a heavy duty chair I went in the park with the dog and the chair spun round on rough ground and threw me out down a slope into a bed of nettles. My hand needed surgery and has never been quite the same since. Wise people learn from other people's experience so I give you a chance to learn from mine.

There are chair-cosies and waterproof covers to wrap round you but no hoods to cover the chair as well as you.

Vehicles Costing £2000 to £3500

Here are the four-wheel electrically-propelled vehicles which bounce up steps as steep as six or even eight inches, have as many as six forward speeds and although the maximum speed is still four miles an hour they can do that uphill. There are two large and two small wheels so no 'kerb-climbers' are necessary. They go very well on rough ground, snow and ice and are strong but not really portable. They *can* be taken apart and folded but it takes a strong person to do it and an estate car to carry the weight. Although you might steer one inside to charge it, they are not indoor chairs. The battery-charger has a cut-out system and if you are not there to switch off when the charge is completed the charger stops input. This is not available on the cheaper chairs. There is also an indicator which tells you how much electricity there is in the batteries and when they need charging.

The *range per battery-charge* is much greater than that claimed for the smaller chairs. Some are said to do 30 miles. The four mile an hour speed limit means you cannot use the full range in one trip in less than eight hours and you'd have to stay overnight to recharge before coming home again. You cannot go on beaches or pebbles in them. If you visit a house which has a drive filled with loose gravel, instead of tarmacadam or concrete, have rescuers standing by to push.

There are some electrically-propelled vehicles which have little fat thick wheels and look like miniature cars. The balloon-like tyres take steps in their stride. There is a hood to cover you and the seat, as well as lights, horn and indicators. They are still four miles an hour pavement vehicles but are bulky for supermarkets and not to be brought indoors unless you have a stately home.

There are two petrol vehicles in this price range.

The Range - Rider

This is the only pedestrian vehicle which will go on gravel, pebbles, wet sand, dry sand, snow, ice, rough country and up and down all pavement edges. It is a three-wheeled vehicle with an engine limited to the legal pavement speed limit. It has three very fat chunky tyres and a battery which starts the four-stroke engine and charges as it runs. You are provided with a trickle-charger to top up the battery if it needs it in winter. The seat is adjustable forwards and backwards and the arms lift up for easy access. You can use a sliding board to get on to the seat from an indoor wheelchair. The handle-bars are as wide as the vehicle so if they go through a gap the rest can follow. The throttle is worked by twisting one handle towards you to go forwards and away from you to go in reverse. When you let go of the throttle the machine stops at once. The seat is over the engine and the petrol tank is behind. You can drive for five hours on a full tank (that is five litres). The engine is noisy and the experience is exhilarating if you put up with the vibration and noise. If you stop for a chat switch off the engine or everyone has to shout. At present it is the only one of its kind and is popular which may, hopefully, bring the price down a bit from £1999 which compares expensively with Hondas and Yamahas. There is a cheaper version called the Outrider but it has a central column over which one leg must be lifted. Fine if you can manage it. It is obviously unsuitable for shops, libraries or anywhere indoors (see illustration on p. 48).

The Nippi

This is a petrol-driven road vehicle and *does* need a road licence and a driving licence. It has the front end and engine of a motor-bike and does 25 miles an hour. Two rear wheels support a platform which has panelling round the front and sides. There is a rear ramp. Lower it, wheel into the Nippi in your wheelchair, raise the ramp, put on your crash helmet, and drive off. You

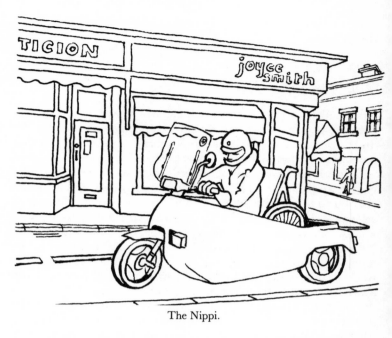

The Nippi.

must stay on the road and use your wheelchair to go into shops or pubs or houses.

Vehicles Costing More than £3500

A car will take you any distance and you can drive it with two hands, one hand or just two feet. Remember to add the cost of your hand-controls to the price. The problem comes when you reach your destination. A hand-propelled chair might limit your shopping or sightseeing when you reach your destination unless you have a sturdy and patient pusher. Electric scooters are manageable. Passers-by can unload those for you, usually.

Vauxhall have solved this by fitting on the driver's door of the Astra an electrically operated arm to hitch the folded hand-propelled wheelchair on to the inner panel. One firm makes a hoist which will lift the driver's wheelchair on to the car roof and slot it under a waterproof cover. It can be fitted to any standard car. There is an electric chair which can be lifted into the driving-seat place in most cars. See or write to *Handicapped Living* (monthly magazine available from any newsagent on order) for information on these. The Elswick Envoy has a rear door and ramp up which you can propel a wheelchair or drive an electric chair. You lock in the wheelchair, fasten the safety-belt and drive off. It's thief proof as there's no driving-seat when you're not in it. There are seats at the rear for two passengers. Ask around—it's amazing what has been invented.

All these vehicles give tremendous independence to the disabled person. They are costly as cars go because they have a limited market. The Mobility Allowance is a great boon. It is not sufficient to buy and run a car but it meets much of the expense. There is a scheme called Motability which takes the whole of your Mobility Allowance all the time, plus a deposit of several hundred pounds, and leases you a car for five years at the end of which time you return it in working order, pay a further deposit and get a new car. The amount of the deposit depends on which car you choose. Most people prefer to manage their own Mobility Allowance and buy a car when they wish to, but don't dismiss Motability without examining it. Get a leaflet from a social worker, the post office, the public library or the DHSS.

Now that more people are living longer and wish to be independent although they are frail, there could be a boom in pedestrian vehicles. I argued in vain to manufacturers in the 1950s that if vehicles for disabled people were designed attractively enough they would sell to a wider market. Most people would like a small, neat, nippy, light-on-fuel, inexpensive means of locomotion. Design needs a new start, scrapping the old 'disability' image. That is why the Range-Rider is so popular. Even babies sitting in prams grin and point with an 'I want one' look on their faces.

Failing to Get Back

There is an element of risk when using any man-made vehicle. The able-bodied walk away from a breakdown to phone the garage and get a bus home. You are stuck until you're repaired. You depend on the kindness and help of passers-by and they have never failed me since 1948. I've been offered cups of tea (very difficult when you can't know when you will be restored to your usable plumbing), a chair on the pavement, an umbrella, a mackintosh, a free phone call and a lift home by various householders near whom I've ground to a halt. I have broken down in every vehicle I've ever driven, except my motorcaravan. Cars can be dealt with by a garage but electric chairs may be 40 or more miles from the repairer. If you are near your home you can disconnect the motor and people will push you, gathering other pushers on the way as the need is seen. If you can stand and get into a car you can lodge your vehicle in the corner of a garage until help can reach it.

There are some sensible precautions you should take whenever you wander far from your own neighbourhood. Have cash for a phone call and a taxi. Make one phone call work and contact one person who will call up a repairer, cancel your appointment, get a taxi, bring you sandwiches or a book to read! Be resigned to a long wait. Keep your cool, don't fuss about your discomfort or your appointment. Be as economical in your demands as possible; don't impose too much. Your rescuer may have an important appointment and feel torn in two directions by his/her needs as well as yours. Be good-humoured and grateful so you don't add to the rescuer's stress. Have the telephone numbers you may need written on card in clearly legible felt-pen, easy to read at night in a phone box without reading glasses. Carry some knitting or a good book so time will pass more quickly.

Here are accounts of some of my own rescues which will, I hope, pass on good advice. If anecdotes annoy, skip them.

Rescue number one

My first breakdown was in an electrically-propelled chair. I was out alone for the first time since becoming disabled. I went to the theatre with a friend who used the bus. On the uphill road home the chair stopped. No lights, no horn. I waved a white hanky at passing cars but roads were not well lit in 1948 and no one saw me. I heard footsteps. Along came a pair of mature ladies with sensible shoes, straight tweed coats and round felt hats, one with a ribbon bow on the front and one with a felt flower on the side. They were eating fish and chips from paper and didn't speak or even appear to see me.

'I wonder if you would help me please? I can't walk and this chair won't go.' In the long pause I went cold with embarrassment. Finally one spoke: '*Whatever* will you think of us? Eating fish and chips from the paper—in the street. *Not* what we are used to, I assure you.' They refused to phone for help and proceeded to push me home. We had regular pauses so they could get their breath back. We chatted and I learnt that this was their Friday night treat, a visit to the cinema in town and a walk home eating fish and chips because no one could see them in the dark. They wouldn't give their names or say where they lived, it was such an adventure! They would fade into the night. And they did. I know no more of them than that.

I got home to a furious family row. There were three roads into town. When I didn't reach home my father walked one way into town and my friend walked another and I had chosen the third. My mother stayed by the phone. When we were assembled again my father declared I was never going out alone again, it wasn't safe. I said I was, I'd a life to live. We learnt the lessons—don't make hasty judgements and assume people aren't willing to help if they hesitate. They've a lot to think about. Secondly, always let people know your route. You owe it to your family not to cause distress and to make it easy for them to cope if you break down. Thirdly, declare your independence, reserve the right to live your life. Fourthly, have change for the phone to make it easy for people to phone for you. There is no substitute for the coin that makes the phone work. To transfer charges is troublesome for a rescuer who may be tongue-tied with embarrassment. Have the phone number clearly written on sturdy card so there is less likelihood of misdialling.

Rescue number two

My next vehicle was a two-stroke petrol-driven three-wheeler and it broke down so often that my pet dachshund used to jump off my knee and run to the passenger door of the breakdown van as soon as it arrived. As one mechanic said when rescuing me for the umpteenth time 'There's not much can go wrong with a two-stroke but what can go wrong always is doing'. It broke down one night as I drove home at pub-closing time from dining with a cousin. I was getting out my phone cash and number card when a worshipper of Bacchus reeled across the pavement and in spite of my warning shout literally fell across my lap. I didn't know what to say. He spluttered, 'Bloody hell, what the devil's this?' I explained carefully and none too hopefully offered my money and my number.

'Nay, lass, I'm too drunk to read that. Who's in if I do ring up?' My mother would be and she'd ring the all-night garage. 'Where do you live?' Two uphill miles away. 'I'll push you'. And he did. I asked him to come in for a rest and a cup of coffee before walking home, back down the hill. 'No, love, there's no need. You've saved me from a right row with the wife, I've sweated myself sober'. Another anonymous rescuer went off into the night and I learnt a valuable lesson—angels of mercy are often well disguised.

Rescue number three

My new car, fresh from its garage servicing, broke down as twilight fell on the A66 in the misty November Lake District. I pulled into a handy lay-by where two Glasgow lorry drivers had just parked their two heavily-laden lorries, having driven their quota of miles for the day. They were going to get warm in the nearest village pub before sleeping all night in their lorries. They diagnosed my problem, a cracked cylinder head, rang for a roadside repair, told the young mechanic what was wrong, sent him back for a new distributor head, stayed till he came back ('He seems a bit slow, we'd best make sure he does it right'), made me a mug of fresh, hot, strong tea, supervised the repair and waved me on my way. They were two splendidly efficient and cheery knight-errants. This is to remind you that winter nights are very cold, so always have a car-rug.

Rescue number four

When my newest electric chair broke down about three months ago in the park I was fortunate to see gardeners working there and I asked the first pair to push me to the second pair. They in turn pushed me to the road and a roundabout where a third pair pushed me round the roundabout and on to my near-by cottage. Flower power! Each gave less than three minutes of time but I got home. Don't ask for more help than you need.

I owe a great debt to my pushers over the last almost 40 years.

7. Work and Play

Speaking chronologically, the first battle is to get the education needed to qualify to become part of the workforce. The Warnock Report and subsequent legislation gave disabled youngsters rights but no one discloses them; you have to discover them. Don't fight for them until you know exactly where to exert pressure, it's too exhausting.

Many authorities are ignoring the law. Suffice it to say that a handicapped child has a right to education in an ordinary school *unless* a panel of experts, including a doctor, psychologist, teacher, physiotherapist and one or both parents, decides that a special school is necessary. This is called 'statementing' a child. In some parts of the country a shortage of psychologists is causing delay. If this causes delay for you it might be worth visiting a psychologist privately to start the ball rolling. Any adaptations your child needs should be made in the ordinary school. Ramps, phonic ears, TV circuits, rails, have all been installed in some state schools to enable the handicapped child to be educated with his/her peers and to experience the world as it will be. You may have to travel further than most to get to a school with the equipment you need but it is your right to have it.

'Re-statementing' your child is possible too. The ordinary school, particularly if it is a large one, may be too exhausting for your child. But remember that all children have problems at some time when trying to fit into school life. If it were not a legal necessity many would opt out—some do! So strike a balance. Encourage always. Offer help. Consult the teacher if there is any sign of disturbance. If school is not viable, educate at home as much as you can. Welcome playmates, supply stimulating play, go out on purposeful visits. Call upon other adults and their skills from time to time. Read *Coping with Your Handicapped Child* in this series.

Further education is not a right in the same way but if you determine to get it you should do so. The Open University is very useful. Local colleges of further and higher education should be examined to see what they offer in the way of courses (and assault-courses such as steps and scattered buildings).

Finding a job

Finding a job has always been hard for disabled people. You must be prepared to accept the fact that you need to be *better* qualified than the able-bodied to get an interview and in order to get the chance to work at all. Your punctuality and attendance must be better than those of anyone else just because they will expect it to be worse. It will be assumed that you are so glad to have a job that you will never want promotion—and you will need as much of it as you can get because you always have extra expenses as this book shows. People serving in shops and cafes at lunchtime assume you're in no hurry and serve you at leisure. People at large assume you don't work and so can't be tired and stressed as they are. You run a car as you need one to get to work and you can afford it if you are working. People take it for granted that you are given a car free by the 'National Health'. This is irritating. I have been told that I'm lucky to be given my car, my electric chair, my crutches, my house, my garage. I need all these and I buy them for myself. The Mobility Allowance came along some years after I was disabled and I have always been very grateful for it and its contribution towards my car costs. You will also find people have a tendency to say with great surprise 'You work?.... How nice.... Aren't you lucky?' Perhaps you are, but you need the work, the status and the money more than the next person. Your living expenses are high.

Job interview

The fact that you need the job so much might give you an air of desperation in an interview which will count against you. Concentrate on setting the interviewers at ease by letting them know things they will be anxious to know but may be embarrassed to ask. They will be worried that your attendance might be poor. You must make a chance to inform them that you go out in all weathers, rain, hail, sleet, snow, fog and gales. Dress well. Make up well and healthily (if you're female, that is). Don't ask for help, move to the set chair and put down sticks or frame or crutches where you can retrieve them unaided. Or park your wheelchair where all can see you and put on the brakes. If a paper is waved at you move in to take it. Smile, speak first and clearly with a 'Hello' or 'Good morning'. Then relax and let them worry about who asks what.

When one of the panel takes a deep breath and begins slowly and carefully with some embarrassment it's fair to assume that they want to know something of your medical condition. Make it easy for them. They will be ignorant, you are an expert in it. Explain clearly and simply. They have a right to know if you go to the hospital from time to time and will need a half-day off for this. You might explain that if you get the job you will be able to pay to visit a consultant and so choose out-of-work time to see him/her. The interviewers owe it to your prospective employer to get to know all they can but they may be genuinely interested in your disability—one may have collected money for research into it for years! Don't be anything but anxious to inform in this. And be cheerful about it. Don't commit yourself to what is not really possible. I was once asked by a head teacher in an interview if I would be able to go round the classroom marking work as children did it. I said the rooms were so overcrowded that one disturbed children if one did this. They had to shuffle chairs to let you pass and this upset their concentration as well as making some nervous of your peering over their shoulder. He didn't agree with me but I wasn't going to promise what would be physically exhausting for me to do when I had a professional reason for my view.

Going to work

When you go to work colleagues will expect you to pull your weight and earn your wages without any help from them. Twenty years ago I would never have said this aloud but over the years I have compared notes with other disabled workers and their experiences match mine, so here goes!

The kindest people, who will be helpful in every way, will not perform kindnesses that are part of the job you are paid for doing. I once had a very painful fall on a school corridor at lunchtime. Just as my leg and spine were stiffening I was due to go up eight steps to mark a register and then come down to go to another room to teach. I asked a colleague whose registration room was next to mine if he would mark my register as well as his own to save me going up and down the steps. The answer was no, and I had to accept it. I once arranged with a colleague to do his dinner duty each week (up and down a flight of steps once) if he would do my corridor duty (up and down the same steps but four times per duty day). He agreed but didn't do the corridor duty and I was reprimanded because it wasn't done. When I explained the exchange I was further reprimanded for messing about with the duty list. When I charged into battle against my colleague he just grinned and said 'It was lovely to have no duty at all for three weeks'. Some men are rough-edged to work with although I thoroughly enjoyed my time as the only female teacher in a large, tough boys' school.

Colleagues will not at first know how to react to you and you have to make your attitude to work clear to them. You have to laugh at an awful lot of bad jokes about disability as people come to terms with it and you train them to ignore it, forget it. People who are made uncomfortable by other people's disabilities have a problem and they need a little unobtrusive help. Be nice to them, don't push towards them, don't prickle. If they are curt or brusque it may be through embarrassment. Help them in small, practical ways—'I'm going there, shall I take it for you?' Hold a door for the person following you. Show you are an equal partner in the working community. It's wise never to ask for help. The sensitive will see your need and won't wait to be asked. The insensitive will feel they're being 'got at' for not offering and the unimaginative will feel that they're earning your money for you. I have not found it helpful or productive to discuss this with the problem-person. However careful one is, it seems to lead to resentment. Try to deal with it indirectly and be adult enough to realise that some people will perhaps just not like you and they have that right!

Hopefully, when the Warnock Report is finally implemented

in schools and disabled pupils are educated and brought up with the able-bodied, these problems will be ironed out and the comments I've made be less necessary.

Unemployed

The 'Protestant ethic' (that work is necessary and good) needs a rethink in late twentieth century unemployment. If you are one of the three million or more unemployed, think about what work is supposed to do that is so good for you, and try to do it for yourself. It gives a disciplined framework to life. You feel better physically if you get up, get dressed, are groomed, go out. The movement is physically stimulating (even exhausting, but practice makes perfect!) and a change of surroundings is a plus. If the surroundings do not please then it's pleasant to be home again. To stick at what is dull or uncongenial (and most people's work gives them a lot of that) gives more flavour to pleasing activities. One finds new ideas and new friends at work so find them by playing positively. Work at playing.

Activities and hobbies

Most hobbies are expensive so go along to a class or a club to see if you like the activity, or like the people who are doing it. You will soon be able to borrow equipment or buy second-hand. It's no use choosing a hobby that doesn't have a band of enthusiasts near you. Find out what opportunities there are in your area. Don't be shy of trying the most unlikely activities, for if the people are lively and likeable it will be fun to go there. Here are ideas that might set you thinking.

Collect things, display things, sell things. Use your home to give simple parties, have a chess championship or find the best player of draughts, ludo, backgammon or scrabble. Join a political party and address envelopes or stand in a local election. Score for the local darts team, cricket team or bowls club. Prompt for the local drama club—a prompt sits still but is needed at all the later rehearsals and at every performance. Seek the chance to become part of some group. Be a mascot. CB Radio is a whole new scene and if you get to know some enthusiasts you may gradually pick up reasonably priced second-hand equipment as others move on to bigger and better sets.

Roll these activities round your mind—Women's Institutes, Townswomen's Guilds, Rotary Clubs, the Lions, darts, indoor bowls, cookery classes and clubs, flower-arranging, growing prize blooms in greenhouse or garden, breeding tropical fish, snooker, singing in a choir, playing bridge, bird-watching, train-spotting, painting pictures, making your own designs of clothes, pottery.

Sports

Sports for the disabled person are growing apace—look at the addresses in the Appendix! Ring up your local sports centres or Town Hall or Education Authority to discover what's going on in your area. Try whatever there is and if you don't like doing the sport that is available see if you enjoy watching others—or train to be a referee!

Pets

Pets are a vexed question as they might involve a lot of work for other people who don't like them. Pets always feel they belong to the person who cares for them so if that isn't you it won't be your pet entirely. Fish in tanks and birds in cages are with you all the time. Cats may or may not be. Dogs delight me and now I live alone I have two. The tiny chihuahua needs little exercise but

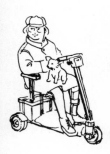

WATCH OUT FOR THE YELLOW SCOOTER!
your
LIBERAL/SDP ALLIANCE CANDIDATE
in the County Council Elections
on 2nd MAY
is trying to talk to as many of the electors as possible.
If you have not yet met her, you will be able to at these times and places:

likes to ride on my knee when I go shopping. The lurcher is a greyhound/deerhound cross and needs several miles a day (in good weather *and* in bad!) as well as a run off the lead in the park or on the beach. One needs a pedestrian vehicle for this (see chapter 6). House-training is not easy and perhaps a friend may help here. The RSPCA often have appealing animals who may be just beyond the destructive puppy stage, under sentence of death unless a home is found for them. Talk to them about what you'd like. The thing about dogs is that they defend you, alert you to visitors, listen to all you say and appear to be devoted to you. If your dog is too excitable it may be the wrong one for you. Be sensible when you choose your dog and train it carefully.

8. Relationships, Strategies and Sex

Every human being spends its life learning to live with itself and others. We emulate, irritate, tolerate, comfort and disturb others as they do us. No one can accurately evaluate the effect he/she has on others, even on those close to them. Those who are successful in relating to others are happy people (and often the unhappy become great and famous!) The single human's struggle, and alliance, with humanity at large is complicated, but not changed, by disability. Disability adds another colour to the weaving but doesn't change the method. Many people have concealed disabilities and in the broadest sense of the word every human has some disability. Being poorer or richer than those around you gives a distorted view of life that starves and shrinks the spirit. Medical conditions, such as diabetes and epilepsy, cause problems to those who develop them but as there is no visible sign of the condition there is no offer of understanding or sympathy or help. In one sense this is fine, as to appear normal is every disabled person's aim. But if a problem requires explanation it can become wearisome.

There is strain for the handicapped in social relationships as many people feel inhibited by others' disabilities. Some approaches are over-hearty and patronising, unfunnily jokey and insulting to the intelligence. One must read the good intention and give marks for effort. Practice will improve the approach so *don't* freeze the person who probably didn't like his/her own words when they fell on the air, anyway. And for those who get it right and come more than halfway towards you, thank God.

You will have to learn to cope with the 'goldfish syndrome' too. You may feel that people are staring. They often are. Remember always that a stare is not intended to be critical or disparaging or distressing. It usually means that the starer is thinking hard about handicap. Should they offer to help? Or just

move in and help? Will you be hurt or offended if they do?
Sometimes the starer has a friend or relative with a similar
handicap to your own and they wonder if what you are using
might be helpful to them. If asked to help they are often very
pleased to do so. Don't waste years, as I did, being cross about
starers. Warm to them, smile.

Remarks that are wide of the mark are best collected into a
jokebook. I once attended a symphony concert in a new red coat.
The audience stood for the National Anthem and I, as usual, felt
that the Queen would understand if I didn't. As the audience
reseated itself I was punched, hard, from behind, on the
shoulder and the word 'Communist!' was hissed in my ear. If
you try to look normal it can only be an achievement when you
succeed.

It is not easy to circulate at social gatherings if you're
handicapped. People can get stuck with you and you with them.
Ask to visit a water-supply (either kitchen or bathroom) and you
will be steered to another area and will make other contacts. Or
ask someone if you can speak to Tom, Dick or Harriet so they
will come to you or you will be shepherded to them. If you sit
feeling stuck you'll look unhappy and won't collect callers.

Habit Forming

This is a vital thing to consider. You'll notice how people become
'set in their ways' as they grow older. Many find a sort of
security in this. Habits, like joints and opinions, stiffen in time
which is why it is courting disaster to marry someone hoping
they will change under your influence. Make a virtue of, make
positive use of this natural tendency to form habits. Make good,
positive habits early in your handicapped living. Discipline
yourself to discover new interests you can take up. Ask all sorts of
people questions about their interests. It makes quiet people
animated and voluble and you may get a chance to cheer them
on as a spectator if you can't join in yourself. Be a good listener as
this rare species is always popular.

Nothing is more boring than an account of illness and pain
and aches, so never give one. If people ask, as they sometimes

do, 'Do you suffer much?' say 'Yes, it's a terrible *bore*' and change the subject. Develop some interest that will make positive use of your time when you're alone. It is good to be alone at times and if your carer knows you can enjoy being alone it eases strain for both of you. Sort collections of photos or letters. Write a history of your family for the younger end of it, write to the papers, have a bird-feeding table outside your window, learn Japanese from a set of tapes, learn to play a recorder or a guitar or a harmonica. Listen to a series of talks or a serial play or reading on the radio. Take up meditation. Design samplers, tapestries, patchwork. Plan a rest from being sociable. Plan menus and shopping trips for you and your carer but don't plan a complicated dish like coq au vin when he/she's had a hard day at work. Design a 'gym' that could help you exercise the bits that can exercise.

Practise pathfinding, ways round obstacles, methods of doing what has not yet seemed possible. At the beginning of this century driving, acting, swimming, sailing and other sports were not considered possible for the disabled person. Pioneers in new machinery and competitors in paraplegic Olympic Games have extended the range of what is thought to be possible for disabled people. When I was recently shown a new, very costly (over £1000) sports wheelchair I was earnestly told, 'You wouldn't stand a chance of a gold medal unless you used this kind. All the medallists at the last games used these'. How to get a gold? Pathfinding, charting new areas of achievement is a painful pursuit as well as exhilarating. It may not suit your temperament or your particular disability. An alternative strategy is to make your room a haven where other people find peace and calm. Be the still centre of the family where there is always a welcome for those who feel in need of one. As families change over time you may be a pioneer at one stage of your life and anchored in harbour at another. Think ahead, make plans, but be flexible. The future may surprise you.

The art of living

Every human has unfulfilled ambitions, hopes and dreams. In Chekhov's play *The Three Sisters*, the girls make drab lives bearable by talking and dreaming of 'When we go to Moscow' and the return to Moscow becomes more and more remote as they grow older and sadder and more ineffectual. It is death to the spirit to dwell on what might have been and it is life and living to set it aside and seek new aims. It is very easy to blame all your unhappiness and all your failure on your disability. It is more honest and more true to admit to yourself that you may never have achieved your goals anyway. Many things turn people aside from their chosen path. Necessary exams may be failed, family break-up may deflect you, a course may be too difficult, you may fall in love with a person who turns you in a new direction, you may be obliged to take a dull, routine job. You may not be selected for what you feel you were born to do. You may dance like a prima ballerina assoluta but if you grow too tall you will not become one. And so on. The art of living is to make strong use of your talents in other ways if you are swept away from your own first choice of lifestyle. You will almost certainly have a harder, more challenging and more interesting life than you expected.

If you have a parent, child, partner, friend who knows you well and whose judgement you respect, get them to assess by putting ticks and crosses against a list of activities, what she/he thinks you will or will not be able to do. See how much they agree with each other and with you. See how many bright ideas can be thought up to enable you to do things that do not seem, immediately, to be possible.

Exercising strong control, as you have to when forming positive habits, means you may find yourself reacting over-dramatically to trifles sometimes. Let fly with gusto *over non-essentials* to let off steam without damaging people around you. But not too often—it's bad-habit-forming.

Breaking the routine

It's wise to build a life that enables you and your carer to have some time apart and some separate activities. Try to arrange one day a week when one of you gets away from the usual routine. The other can be alone or with a friend. (Many people find being alone a healing change but if you don't, don't arrange to be!)

Once a week have a meal out, at a pub, transport cafe or the Ritz, together or separately, even if it means very cheap meals at home next day. One evening a week try local evening classes (which are often free for the disabled person). You can go to the centre together and then attend different classes. It gives you a chance to make new friends and if you don't enjoy car maintenance give woodcarving a go next session. On Sundays go, together or separately, to a church or chapel or Quaker meeting. Choose the latter if you like silence and the former if you enjoy a good sing. This is not to suggest that you become a believer if you are not, but to point you to a place where you can expect to meet caring people, break away briefly from home relationships and make new contacts. It also gives the spirit a breathing-space. There may be weekly discussion groups, a hall you could hire for a fund-raising effort. Holidays apart can be arranged through special agencies (see the address in the Appendix). It's good to be homesick or to look forward to going again next year.

Role-swapping

This is often necessary and imposes a great strain on relationships. If he has always done the home-decorating and she now has to, his obvious doubts will depress her and make her failure more likely. Try to get tips and confidence helping a friend at first, away from the critical gaze of the expert. If he has to take over the cooking, he needs to practise simple dishes with step by step instruction. Teach each other gently and patiently. Make haste slowly. Begin with easy things. Lest anxiety and stress should flare into a row, ask in a friend you both respect to act as a referee if necessary (or to maintain your good manners with each other!) Embark on totally new recipes so that you can't compare the new cook's version with the old cook's version. If you've never had curry at home, now's the time to try it. TV cookery programmes are most helpful as in the 20 minute programme nothing too complicated is attempted. You can watch, make notes, then try it at the weekend.

Don't let the nuts and bolts of running a house strain relationships to breaking-point. A war against dust and dirt, pots and pans shouldn't be allowed to cause human casualties. It should be realised that there is nothing more stressful to someone who kept house than sitting helpless while a myriad small jobs beckon. It may be possible to trade skills with a neighbour. You get some shopping for her as you exercise the electric chair while she dusts through the house for you. Mending, sewing on buttons, peeling vegetables and preparing fruit were all things I hated and they were dropped into my lap to 'give you something to do' when I much preferred needlepoint. Perhaps that led to my iron determination to get a job. If you trade skills you have the satisfaction of seeing your home smile after someone has tickled it with a duster, but a word of warning. Beware how you tie yourself down to a regular weekly appointment. It may become irksome, you may not always feel sociable on Fridays at nine a.m. If the arrangement is for a different time and/or day each week it is easier to space it out so it will not turn sour. You may forget to be thankful that the difficult-for-you job is done and begin to be critical of the doer's way of doing it, or of her/his gossip. Rescue the friendship; rethink the dusting. A regular weekly arrangement may give you a feeling of order and security. I often felt trapped by such arrangements. Loss of spontaneity in life is the thing I felt keenly in being disabled. Arrangements invariably have to be made to have side doors opened, parking places saved, the level access theatre tickets booked, so impulse outings are not possible.

Sex

This century has seen a revolution in attitudes to sex. It could be claimed that we're better at dealing with sex than we are at dealing with death. Before Freud we got it the other way round. Once the great unmentionable, sex is now open to frank discussion. People's sexuality plays a prominent part in advertisements, films, plays, books, magazines, newspapers and TV programmes. In this area we learn from fiction, 'life imitates art', because previous generations were more inhibited than we are in an age of ever-growing frankness. Remember that attitudes have changed, sex hasn't. Sadly, sex seems to have become yet another area where there is success and failure.

Prowess is admired and young people feel they should become experienced and 'good' at it. The acceptance of divorce, cohabitation and a certain amount of promiscuity means that the interesting struggle to build a lasting, strong and tough relationship is abandoned part-way along the journey towards it and much suffering results. Handicap or disability can be a severe strain on relationships. You are more likely to be tired, in pain, limited physically. You will feel as though you appear less attractive although attraction is deeper than that. Relationships that are strong will grow powerfully. Those that are weak may strengthen or fracture. You face important issues together. If you have a partner now is the time for tenderness, closeness, cuddling and physical contact. Now is the time for honest expressions of love and fear.

Sex therapists and sex counsellors have come into existence to deal with problems in sexual relationships, so disabled people should remember that they are not alone in having problems with sexual performance. Also remember the infinite variety in human relationships, give and take, swings and roundabouts, negotiated compromises, and be aware of this, not afraid of it. I well remember the shout of laughter from a group of women friends at a coffee morning when one said: 'I was thrilled when I'd reached the change of life. I told Henry, that's the end of all that. And you know, it was such a relief not to have to pretend to enjoy it any more'. She had an apparently warm relationship with her husband, two affectionate sons, an attractive personality and the marriage survived with no discernible tensions. Don't let writers overplay the sex card. Humans, their needs and their joys, are of infinite variety.

It has been suggested that disabled people should be encouraged or even helped to have casual sex so that they do not miss out on what life has to offer. This surely debases sex. Sex should be part, and only part, of an ever-developing relationship with another person. Unless sex reinforces the respect and tenderness each feels for the other it is merely a form of physical exercise (which was assumed by boys' public schools for many years when they promoted games as ideal pastimes for adolescent boys), and other forms of exercise are available.

Anyone who marries a disabled person is obviously committed to that person and will be ready to tackle problems with courage and confidence.

The mass media 'lead us into temptation' in many areas of life. They try to teach us to want central heating, electric washers, perfect marriage partners, dyed hair, leather furniture, and they show sexual attraction as the highway to bliss. It is not as important to ordinary people in their daily lives as the admen try to make us believe. Use the energy somewhere else if you have to. Use the steam to drive another engine. Be creative! Writing romantic novels may bring enough money for you to live quite happily without sex if sex doesn't work out for you.

9. Lifting Bodies and Spirits

Notes for Carers

If you have to lift the body here is some practical advice.

The Right Equipment

This is more than half the battle. Get it and get used to using it before you feel the strain. There are special beds and baths which tilt, operated electrically. There are hoists which can be worked by an attendant or by the patient to transfer people to and from beds, cars or baths. Look at the addresses in the Appendix to which you can write for a comprehensive list of what you need. If you explore what is available it is easier for Social Services to help you.

Sliding boards are easy to use and to make. The board is slippery on top because you've sand-papered it and given it one

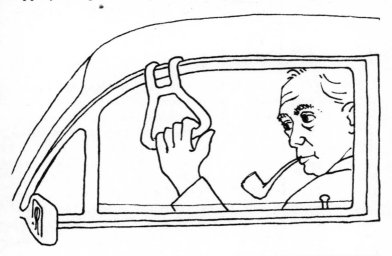

or two coats of polyurethane varnish. You've done the edges as well so they're smooth, too. Underneath you've stuck a rubber mat or strips of rubber or plastic to make it stable. For extra safety you nail a strip of wood underneath at each end so that the board lodges firmly over the side of the wheelchair, the bath, or the car seat. The exact measurement depends on the sizes of the car, bath, wheelchair and patient. If the user puts it in place and puts it aside, it needs to be light to handle. But it also needs to be able to take the weight, regularly. To save carrying it about, have several—one each in bedroom, bathroom and garage. Look for thrown-away tables, wardrobes or drawers for usable wood. A 'monkey-pole' (see picture p. 33) helps you to heave up or down the bed, or up off the bed while a sheet is changed. If you can take weight on your hands and arms to move up and down the bed you will probably find your undercarriage drags on the bed and this isn't good. Nail D-shaped door handles on to blocks of wood three inches deep and you'll get extra clearance by gripping these as you move or lift. Another way of getting extra lift is to tie together several same-size books with broad tape or ribbon. Grip the books with your fingers and thumbs slotted under the tie. Never drag a patient up and down as sheets rub and injure the skin. There is a Duffield Patient Lift Belt which can be used under the patient to prevent rubbing.

Heave-Ho, Muscle-Power

Half-an-hour with a good physiotherapist teaching you how to lift is most worthwhile. You must beware of back injury, as once acquired it's very hard to lose. Take care of your back because there's no substitute for it. The leg muscles are the strongest in the body, most capable of taking strain and weight. Bend and use hips, knees, ankles and keep the back straight. Never try to give a big swing or heave, it's too much strain on the spine. Don't pull on the patient's arms and legs as it's a painful strain on the joints and a patient in pain is harder to move. Patient and carer are a team and must work together. Firm confidence is the key, not speed. Never lift or pull or push if the patient can lift, pull or push him/herself.

Learn the finger grasp, double-wrist grasp, double-forearm grasp, palm-to-palm thumb grasp from physiotherapist or nurse. Learn how to use the patient's ability to rock sideways or forwards and backwards as a means of gradually shifting position or heaving on to the feet.

If a disabled person should fall, make them as comfy and warm as you can and leave them to recover from the shock (it's hateful to be heaved on to one's feet while still breathless and people always rush to set one to rights in this way) while you get assistance in case you need it. Always check the stability of a chair, if it's a wheelchair putting on *both* brakes, before lifting a patient on to it. If a walking disabled person becomes unstable because of a sudden gust of wind, patch of ice, an indoor rug, mat or wet lino, never seize an arm—it's as dangerous as if someone seized an able-bodied person's leg without warning. Anyone who uses crutches, a walking frame or sticks is walking on their hands and arms. Don't get hold of them. Stand by so he/she can seize your arm because you will give stronger support than the stick/frame/crutch. Alternatively you might hold the waist to keep the unsteady walker on balance, but only if you're aware of their particular weakness and can counteract it.

Wheelchairs

When the user is propelling a wheelchair, never take over from behind without warning. Most people hold the tyre as well as the propelling circle (which is slippery and too narrow to grip easily). This means that finger-ends are dangerously near spokes. If the wheel is suddenly spun fast without warning, nails are torn and finger-ends can be wrenched or bruised.

When you're navigating steps, tilt the chair back on to its big wheels so that the user is gazing at the sky or the ceiling. There are two reasons. One is that this keeps the user firmly in the chair. The second reason is that the big wheels will bounce up or down a step and little wheels will not, so put the little wheels in the air out of the way. If small wheels meet a doormat at speed the user can be tossed out!

Folding wheelchairs works if you follow this plan. Pull up the footrests first or they will jam into each other and lock when the

81

chair is half folded. To fold up the chair hold the centre back of the seat with one hand and the centre front of the seat with the other and lift up. Pushing the sides together is a waste of energy as it does not work. Open the chair by pressing down on both sides of the seat. Don't press the armrests although it's tempting because they're easier to reach than the seat-sides. And when you press the seat-sides and the chair does open watch out for your fingers—the armrests catch them as the chair opens out.

Lifting The Spirits

Disabled people can tyrannise those around them, cashing in on sympathy. So can carers. It's unwise and counter-productive. Disabled persons often have untapped energy which becomes a vital force in a power struggle. Beware. Don't be a doormat but don't start a hurtful fight that neither of you will be able to forget. And don't take decisions for each other. Establish firmly that handicapped people do all they can for themselves. If in the early stages too much help is given it is hard and difficult to withdraw it later. It is better for the disabled person to be stretched, exercised and as active as possible by doing all that he/she can do even if it takes a long time. Also it is better for *both* that dependency should be reduced as much as possible. The more you limit your contact the easier it is for someone else to take over for a time if the carer needs a holiday or a stay in hospital.

A disabled body doesn't stop the mind working. Avoid taking decisions for disabled people. Don't manage medicines and bedtimes as though you were dealing with a child. It is offensive to the disabled person and very embarrassing for others. Never say 'He' or 'She' when John or Betty is right there and should be acknowledged as a person.

When you're tired, say so. Sit down with a cup of tea and put up your feet for a while. Honesty is best and most practicable. When you've a problem discuss it together. Acknowledge your dependency on the person you care for. Use his/her skills and experience to get advice on your work problems. If you can, get help with some of the cleaning or gardening so that you have some time to sit and talk.

If you have a row remember that your opposite number can't storm out and bang the door. You can. It's frustrating not to be able to. If possible, always have rows over small things. You can laugh about them afterwards. The big things matter too much in your case. Never carry a grudge overnight, your time together is too precious. Have a drink, clear the air, kiss and make up.

When offered help always try to take up the offer in some way. People are hurt and they withdraw if their help is refused. You have denied them and judged them useless. Think hard to find a way to use their help. Ask them to collect dry-cleaning, an order at the butcher's, return library books, find a shop that has cotton nightwear, find a gardener for a short time each week for you.

Disabled people can be just as crabby, unreasonable, bad tempered, edgy and mean as the rest of the human race. So can carers. And you have more than most to try your patience. So you both have to exercise more control than most people do. In the disabled/carer relationship each needs to be very tender of the other's fragile dignity and self-respect. Pain, mental or physical, does not improve anyone's tolerance. Try to remove small irritations. Remember that your fear, anxiety, sadness will rub off on to each other. Depression and anger must be well controlled and safely and constructively discharged if relationships are to thrive and survive. Share jokes. Laugh as much as you can. Give and take warmth and affection. Make the most of every minute of your lives together. Be apart at times to recharge the batteries. If this sounds very demanding never mind—surprise yourselves and each other. Human beings have tremendous capabilities and powers lying dormant within them.

10. Experiences

The Stroke-Victim's Wife

'It was four years ago… it was an absolute nightmare. We'd only just removed to a bigger house in the country with an acre of garden. The boys were seven and nine years old, settling in to their new school. George was sent to Eastern Europe by his firm for 10 days. On his second day there he had an awful stroke. He was only 42. They treated him extremely well. Did all the tests very thoroughly and sent full reports home with him. He was in hospital here for eight months. I've never felt such utter despair. He hadn't to be worried. The prognosis was very poor. He must have no stress. Oddly enough, the only thing that kept me going was the feeling that things just couldn't get any worse. Because we'd only just moved into the area I was too far away from my old friends and neighbours to have daily contact with them and I missed that. The new neighbours were really very kind but it wasn't quite the same. I didn't know them well enough to cry to them, if you see what I mean.

George came home after eight months using two sticks and only able to walk a very few slow steps. We had a wheelchair. He'd always done the driving but I'd had to take that over, I needed the car to visit the hospital. His work had been very demanding and we were warned he mustn't go back to it. The firm was quite good. We got a lump sum and a very small pension, lucky to get that. We'd had good insurance fortunately and I made a little extra money indexing books. One problem was how to protect George from stress. I was under tremendous stress—and how!—with George to care for, the boys, the house, the driving, the garden, the shopping, taking George to hospital for treatment, indexing, managing the money… The physiotherapy was such a help as it gave George something to think about and work at between treatments… One day we had a blazing row about how much milk I'd ordered and that's when I decided it was time we cleared the air a bit, if you see what I mean. I let George know how much worry I'd had and what decisions I'd had to make. He took it quite well. I didn't nag or

whine but I let him know something of what I'd been through....
It was good that we'd always had a joint hobby, playing piano
duets and two-piano works. We did this every day after he came
home from hospital. At first he could only play 'Chopsticks' but
now we're back on to Mozart...

I used to work off my aggression on the garden. I'd go out
there and dig, and wrestle with unwanted shrubbery and burn
the rubbish and the boys helped with all that and we talked as we
did it. I prayed a lot as well, I'm a Christian but George isn't.
George said he was trying to find the right balance between
physical and intellectual effort in coping with his speech
problems. Relaxation and movement, discipline and control of
mind and body were his preoccupations... and we're so thrilled
with his progress, he's worked so hard at it and he's done so
much better than we dared to hope. Four years after the stroke he
only uses one stick when he's very tired. The wheelchair hasn't
been out of the garage for over a year. I don't think he thought I
would be able to cope as I did and I think he respects me more,
funnily enough. And I feel deeply chuffed. And so thankful that
we've come through it all, together. We seem to have learnt a lot
about life and about each other...'

The Disabled Wife

'We were both working, our daughter was in the sixth form and
our son was doing 'O' levels. My husband's a teacher and I
worked in an office. Everything was fine. Then I had a tumour
on the knee and it was malignant, so the leg had to be amputated.
The next 18 months I can't bear to think about. You get by. You
live one day at a time and try not to look forward because you
don't know how things'll work out. Sometimes when I was
depressed I used to get really mad with the family. They were
super, really good to me, they seemed to understand. I'd never
have coped without them.

The first artificial leg was a mess. It needed so many
adjustments they finally started all over again. The second leg
was better but it took a long time to get used to it. I fell quite a bit
and it's embarrassing when you're out shopping and you
suddenly fall over. My mother always came with me when I went
shopping at first because she worried about me. It was mean of
me, but I often thought I'd be better on my own because she

fussed and worried more than I liked. But she was ever so good to me.

I always had my hair done regularly and took care to wear nail-varnish and make-up. I didn't want to let myself go.

We had the car adapted with a hand control so I could drive it, but my husband needed it for work, he'd a long way to travel, and we couldn't afford two cars. I've got a part-time job in my old office and I'm saving up to get a small car. I can't get a mobility allowance, one leg amputation isn't enough. And I wouldn't use an invalid chair because I don't want to look disabled.

I was so looking forward to getting my artificial leg but it wasn't easy to manage with it. I thought it would be a great step forward but it felt like ever so many steps back. The harness is so heavy. I'm not sure how helpful it is to read books and see films about real-life people like Douglas Bader. I found shopping, especially supermarket shopping, was exhausting and a lot of the time frightening as well. If my husband came to help we were there at the busy times and it was worse. I felt that flying a plane or being heroic would be a lot easier than washing and cleaning and shopping. The family were ever so helpful but they were out at school all day and I was there in the house with the work waiting to be done and I couldn't leave it to pile on them when they came home. It's very hard to do housework when you're disabled. We're moving soon to an easier house with a bigger, better-equipped kitchen as we've decided it's more important than a second car for me. We need to win the pools to get a car for me.

It's been very hard on all of us, on my husband and son and daughter too, they've been marvellous to me... Without them I'd never have coped and when I say that, they say "we're all right Mum, it could have been so much worse" and it could!'

The Single Disabled Career Woman

'I had a good job and my own house and I was engaged to be married. Then I was in a car accident and had two years in hospital having surgery and treatment, at the end of which I was in a wheelchair. My fiancé was a bit—a lot—long-winded about it but he quite determinedly faded from the scene. I had sold my house as it was no good to me in a wheelchair. I couldn't live with my parents because they were too protective, they worried too much. I bought a bungalow and had it adapted. I wanted to get back to work and live an independent life. There was no unemployment then but getting a job was damned hard. Finding a work-place without steps was the first hurdle. I got work eventually because I had a useful specialty.

You need extra cash in all sorts of areas. Your car has to be reliable, you can't run an old banger. Clothes wear out quickly when you use a wheelchair, the sleeves especially catch and rub. Ground-floor theatre seats are expensive. Holidays cost more because you need a hotel with a lift big enough to take a wheelchair and with porters, and such hotels are more costly than smaller hotels.

I prefer holidays alone because when you're alone people talk to you freely. It may be the wheelchair that helps them to approach you but I've picked up some rare characters on both sides of the Atlantic.

I had a motor-home at one point and I'd recommend that to disabled drivers. That was first class. Park in a camping site and slide through to the back of the motor-home where you have bed, cooker, mod. cons. It was the most trouble-free holiday home one could imagine. I could't afford it after I retired but I'd have another tomorrow if I came into money!

I've always paid for help in the house. You can't have a home-help if you're not in the house and that's reasonable enough. Shopping's sheer hell in supermarkets but getting in and out of half-a-dozen smaller shops is also very difficult. If you work you can only go when it's crowded and hard to park. A wheelchair and an erratic trolley are terrible awkward. You can't ask other people to shop for you because they don't know what alternative to get if something isn't available. I like to be independent and fend for myself. I feel it very strongly. I dread losing my autonomy. All people do, but disabled people feel it more than most, I think.

Airports are well geared to dealing with wheelchairs and so are trains and stations as long as you let them know beforehand. You have to be well organised and I can certainly say I'm that. I've had to be. I think I've coped with disability very well. A good job, a good home, good holidays. But I desperately wish it hadn't happened, to be absolutely honest. I see no nobility whatsoever in suffering. I'm sure if we're honest we'd all say the same.'

The Disabled Man Alone

'Well, I don't know if I can be helpful, but here goes. I worked in London, in and around Parliament. I'd separated from my wife and bought her a house so she was settled. Our elder son was at Cambridge and the younger one away at school. I had a flat in Westminster and I went jogging every morning as I was getting a bit flabby. I was 47. Then I had this severe stroke and brain surgery. My right side was paralysed and I lost my speech. It took five years of really hard work to learn to speak again as well as I do now. I can walk with a stick and drive a car though my right arm and hand are useless.

I got a lump sum and small pension from my employers and they gave me the Granada which had been my company car. I sold that and my flat. So what to do next? I decided to move north as houses are cheaper here. I live in a small country town with about 8000 inhabitants. I get a mobility allowance. I bought a small house and a car. I have physiotherapy at the local hospital and I have a home-help. I eat out a lot as it's not expensive here. I used to be a good cook but I can't get used to working in a kitchen with only one usable hand in spite of gadgets. My left hand always expects my right hand to cooperate and it can't. Funny feeling. I go to local history classes and I joined the local bird-watchers' club. I fell in my garden watching birds and broke my leg but I was well cared for in hospital and the leg healed well. I've got to know quite a few people. I live a totally different life now and I'm truly very happy. It's good to be out of the rat-race though when I was in it I thought it was the right and proper place to be. Now I feel differently.'

The Disabled Woman's Husband, Looking Back.

'My wife was lame. She'd had polio when she was nine. She used two sticks and wore two callipers. She was a grand lass. We'd five children and they all turned out well. I was a school-caretaker and we needed all the brass I could earn but getting extra brass meant doing overtime and I couldn't help her as much as I'd've liked with the children. And now, looking back, I wish I'd been with her more. She died just four months after I'd retired. We had good times together but I want her with me now when I'm not working. We couldn't ever afford a car, out of the question. I

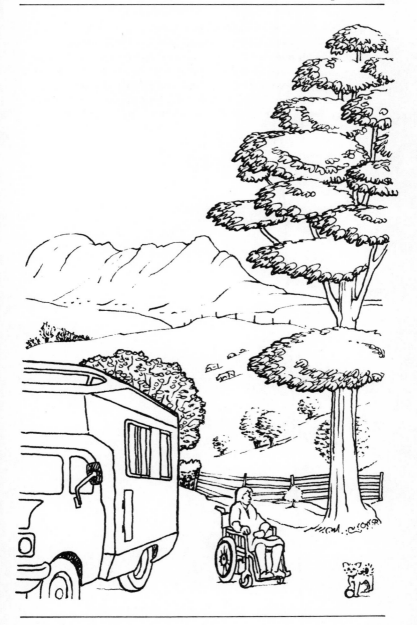

wish they'd had these little electric things then. I could have got her one of those and we'd've been able to go out together, me walking with her. But we right enjoyed our family—they're all over England now. Two of the lads went in the Air Force and they've both travelled all over the world. You shouldn't have favourites but my lass in Sheffield's the one I like staying the best. She's just like her mother and wonderful with her children.'

Useful Addresses

Royal Association for Disability and Rehabilitation
25 Mortimer Street
London W1N 8AB
Tel. 01-637 5400

Gives advice and information on education, employment, mobility and access. Books are available too.

Disabled Living Foundation
380-384 Harrow Road
London W9 2HU
Tel. 01-289 6111

Has a comprehensive display of, and brochures about, aids and equipment, including stair-lifts, electric and self-propelled wheelchairs, bathroom, kitchen, bedroom and toilet aids. An appointment should be made to see these. Experts are there to advise.

Disability Alliance
25 Denmark Street
London WC2H 8NJ
Tel. 01-240 0806

Produces in November each year a book about all the benefits to which people may be entitled.

Scottish Council on Disability
Princes House
5 Shandwick Place
Edinburgh EH2 4RG
Tel. 031-229 8632

An information and advice centre.

Scotland's Disabled Aids Shop
45 Carlyle Avenue
Hillington Industrial Estate
Glasgow G52 4XX
Tel. 041-882 9946

In the mornings, viewing by appointment only. Open to the general public in the afternoons. All aids, including plumbing and wheelchairs, can be ordered for immediate delivery.

Equipment for the Disabled
Dept 355
Mary Marlborough Lodge
Nuffield Orthopaedic Centre
Windmill Road
Headington
Oxford OX3 7LD
Tel. 0865 64811

A series of reference books published by the Oxfordshire Health Authority on behalf of the DHSS.

Special Equipment and Aids for Living (SEQUAL)
Block 178
Milton Trading Estate
Abingdon
Oxon. OX14 4ES

Has a full-time welfare staff and a visiting officer. Publishes a quarterly magazine *Possibility*.

Possum Users Association
27 Thames House
140 Battersea Park Road
London SW11

COMMUNICATION AIDS CENTRES are to be found at:

Boulton Road
West Bromwich
West Midlands

Royal Victoria Infirmary
Queen Victoria Road
Newcastle upon Tyne
Tel. 091-232 5131

Speech Therapy Dept.
Frenshay Hospital
Bristol
Tel. 0272 565656

MONEY FOR RESEARCH is raised by these special groups:

Action for Research into Multiple Sclerosis
Central Middlesex Hospital
Acton Lane
London NW10 7NS
Tel. 01-453 0142

Arthritis and Rheumatism Council for Research
41 Eagle Street
London WC1R 4AR
Tel. 01-405 8572

International Spinal Research Trust
Strand House
New Fetter Lane
London EC4A 1AD

Action Research for the Crippled Child
Vincent House
North Parade
Horsham
West Sussex RH12 2DA
Tel. 0403 64101

Sportsmen Pledged to Aid Research into Crippling Diseases
is also at the above address.

SOURCES OF INFORMATION ABOUT SPECIFIC PROBLEMS

National Ankylosing Spondylitis Society
6 Grosvenor Crescent
London SW1X 7ER
Tel. 01-235 9585

Chest, Heart and Stroke Association
Tavistock House
Tavistock Square North
London WC1H 9JE
Tel. 01-387 3012

65 North Castle Street
Edinburgh EH2 3LT
Tel. 031-225 6963

National Association for Deaf, Blind and Rubella Handicapped
311 Gray's Inn Road
London WC1X 8PT
Tel. 01-278 1005

Friedreich's Ataxia Group
Burleigh Lodge
Knowle Lane
Cranleigh
Surrey GU6 8RD
Tel. 0483 272741

Haemophilia Society
123 Westminster Bridge Road
London SE1 7HR
Tel. 01-928 2020

Headway: National Head Injuries Association
200 Mansfield Road
Nottingham
Tel. 0602 622382

Multiple Sclerosis Society of Great Britain and Northern Ireland
286 Munster Road
Fulham
London SW6 6AP
Tel. 01-381 4022/4025 or 01-385 6146/7/8

Muscular Dystrophy Group of Great Britain and Northern Ireland
Nattrass House
35 Macaulay Road
London SW4 0QP
Tel. 01-720 8055

Parkinson's Disease Society
36 Portland Place
London W1N 3DG
Tel. 01-323 1174

British Polio Fellowship
Bell Close
West End Road
Ruislip
Middlesex HA4 6LP
Tel. 0895 675515

Spastics Society
12 Park Crescent
London W1N 4EQ
Tel. 01-636 5020

Scottish Council for Spastics
22 Corstorphine Road
Edinburgh EH12 6HP
Tel. 031-337 9876

Association for Spina Bifida and Hydrocephalus
22 Upper Woburn Place
London WC1H 0EP
Tel. 01-388 1382

Scottish Spina Bifida Association
190 Queensferry Road
Edinburgh EH4 2BW
Tel. 031-332 0743

Spinal Injuries Association
76 St James's Lane
London N10 3DF
Tel. 01-444 2121

Sexual and Personal Relationships of the Disabled
286 Camden Road
London N7 0BJ
Tel. 01-607 8851/2

Publishes leaflets and a regular bulletin. Gives advice and counsels disabled people.

ESPECIALLY FOR CARERS

Association of Carers
1st Floor
21-23 New Road
Chatham
Kent ME4 4QJ
Tel. 0634 813981

Supplies information and publications.

Holiday Care Service
2 Old Bank Chambers
Station Road
Horley
Surrey RH6 9HW
Tel. 0293 774535

SPORTS OPPORTUNITIES FOR DISABLED PEOPLE

British Sports Association for the Disabled
Hayward House
Barnard Crescent
Aylesbury
Buckinghamshire HP21 8PT
Tel. 0296 27889

Scottish Sports Council
Development Officer for Persons with Disabilities and Handicaps
1 St Colme Street
Edinburgh EH3 6AA
Tel. 031-225 8411

Riding for the Disabled Association
Avenue R
National Agricultural Centre
Kenilworth
Warwickshire CV8 2LY
Tel. 0203 56107

National Anglers' Council, Committee for Disabled Anglers
11 Cowgate
Peterborough PE1 1LZ
Tel. 0733 54084

Archery for Disabled People
7 New Street
Shifford
Bedfordshire SG17 5BW

British Disabled Waterski Association
Warren Road
The Warren
Ashtead
Surrey KT21 25N

British Ski Club for the Disabled
Corton House
Corton
Warminster
Wiltshire BA12 0SZ

Specialist Wheelchairs for Sports
Hugh Steeper (Roehampton) Ltd.
237-239 Roehampton Lane
London SW15 4LB

Disabled Drivers' Association
Ashwellthorpe
Norwich NR16 1RX

Disabled Drivers' Motor Club
1a Dudley Gardens
Ealing
London W13
Tel. 01-840 1515

HAND CONTROLS FITTED IN YOUR OWN GARAGE TO CARS, TRACTORS, MOBILE HOMES, ETC.

Alfred Bekker
The Green
Langtoft
Driffield YO25 0TF
Tel. 0377 87276

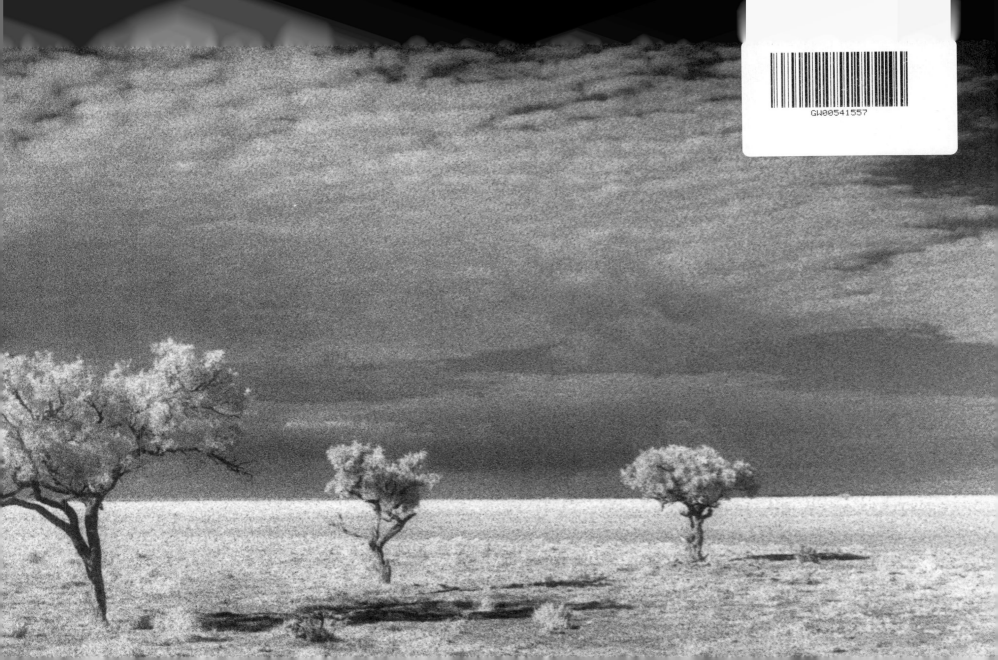

A Day in the Outback

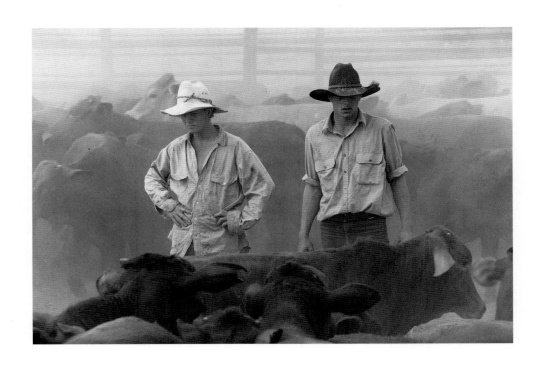

Mark Coombe

THE OUTBACK ... What is it?

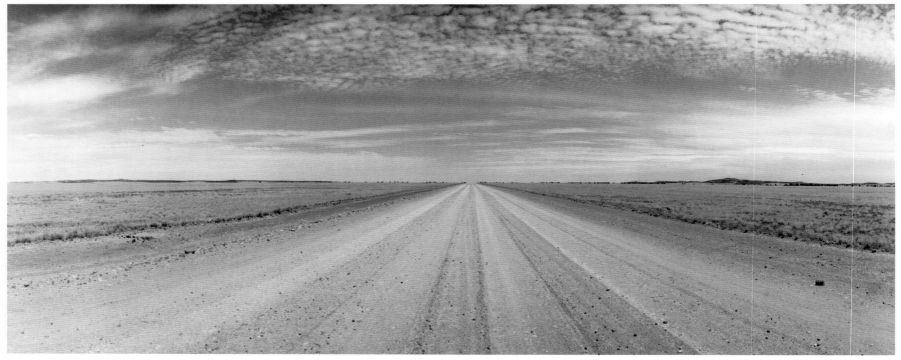

The road to Birdsville, 150km west of Windorah

THE OUTBACK ... Where is it?

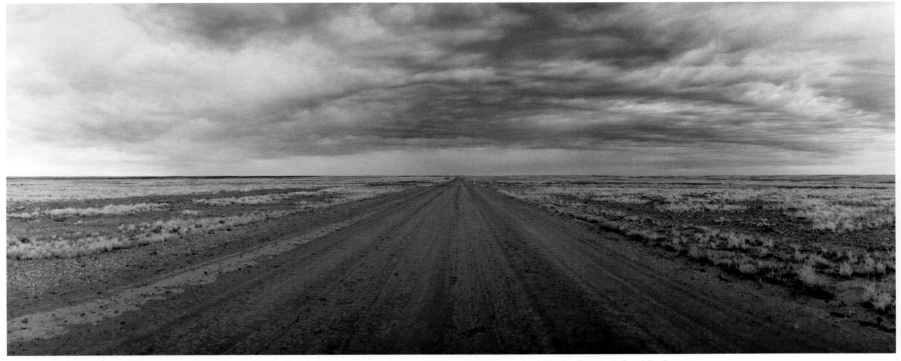

Another Outback road, 15km north of the South Australian border between Durrie Station (100km east of Birdsville) and Cordillo Downs

THE OUTBACK

The term "Outback" is hard to define, and I guess everyone's idea of what it is, and where it is may vary somewhat. I'm sure someone from a big city would have a very different opinion as to what the Outback is compared to someone from a small country town or an outback property.

For me the Outback means; wide-open spaces, long straight roads and dusty tracks, spectacular sunsets, long hard working days, friendly people and isolation.

There isn't a line that you can stand on and say this is where the Outback begins or ends. To me it's a feeling you get when travelling. You reach a certain point when you feel you are in the "Outback". It's hard to describe but you just know when you are there.

This book shows what is happening at any time of the day on any number of different Outback properties.

I hope this book will leave you with an insight into the daily lives of the people working in the Outback. Along the way you will get to experience the beauty of Australia.

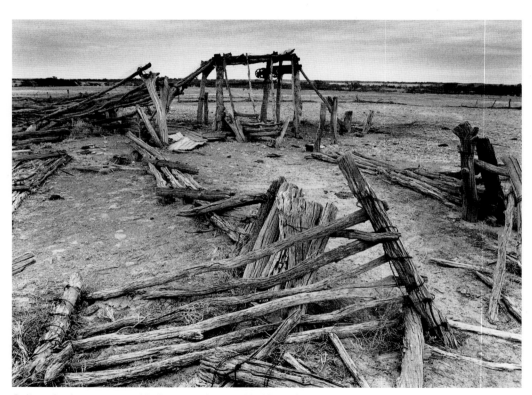

Relics of a bygone era, old sheep yards near Haddons Corner

Facing Page: A twisted Gidgee tree somewhere on Tobermorey Station shows the harshness of the Outback (Infra-red photograph)

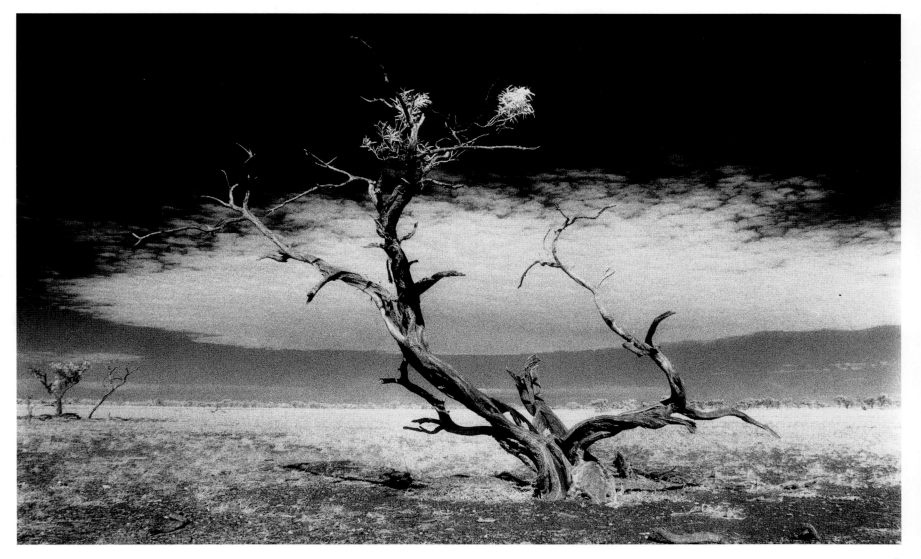

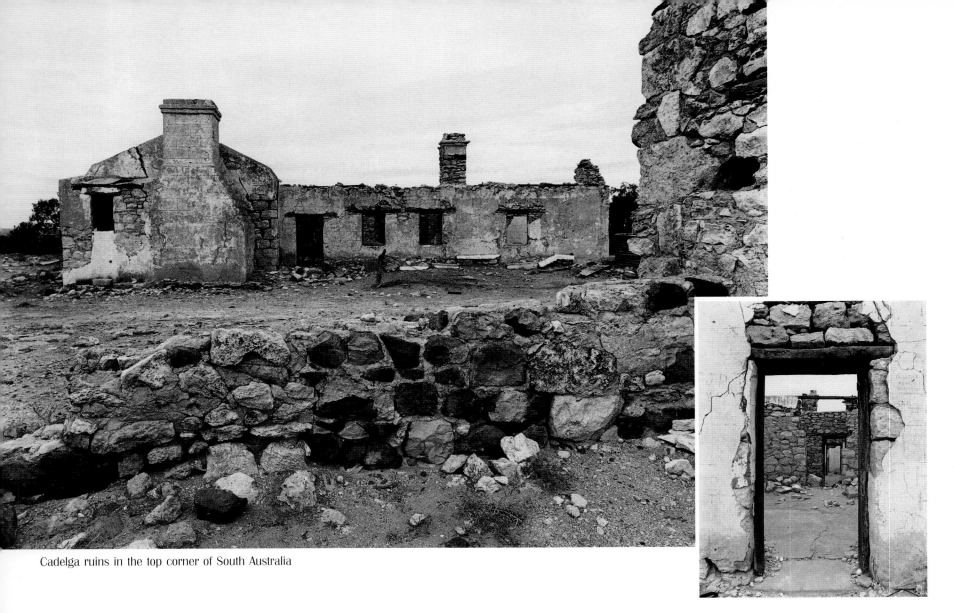

Cadelga ruins in the top corner of South Australia

6

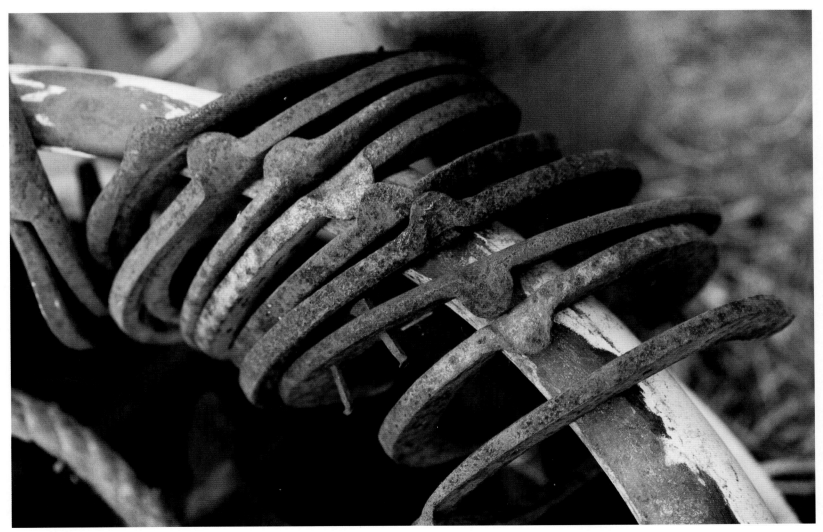

Rusty shoes

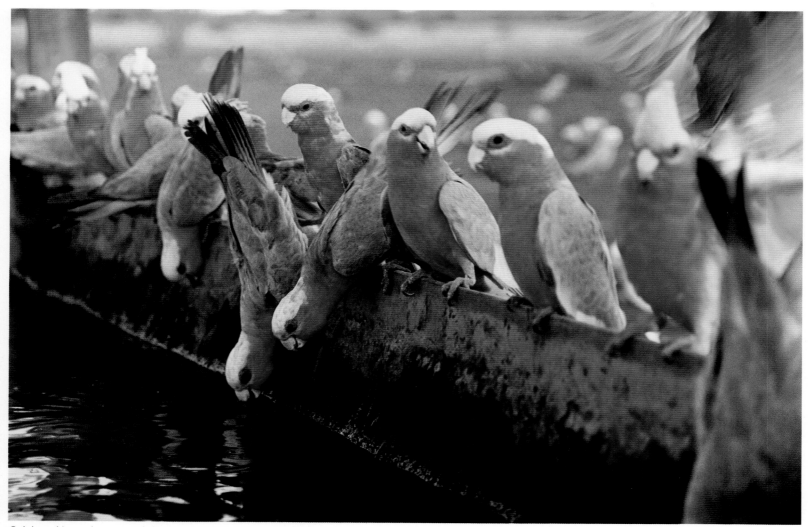
Galahs taking advantage of the most valued commodity in the outback ... water

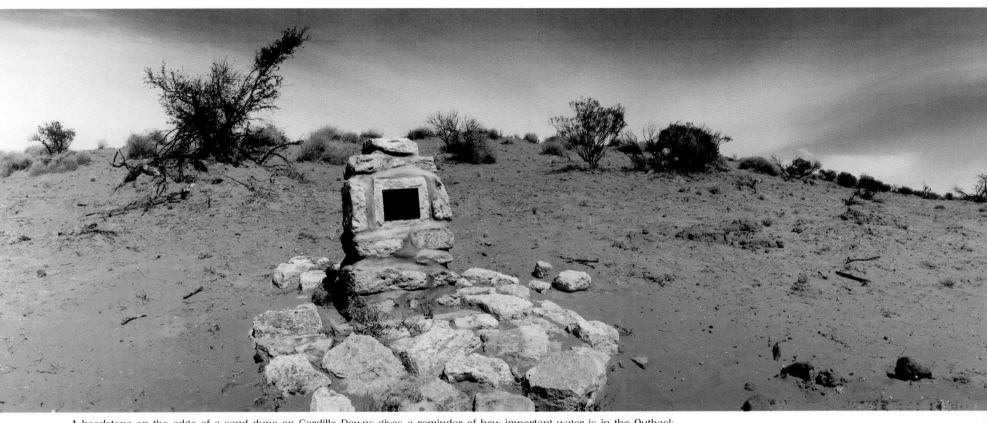

A headstone on the edge of a sand dune on Cordillo Downs gives a reminder of how important water is in the Outback

The headstone reads: "In loving memory – John Hisgrove Died 30/10/1896 Aged 55. Perished for want of water. Had been working at Haddon Downs and Arrabury during shearing. Erected by his descendants 1995".

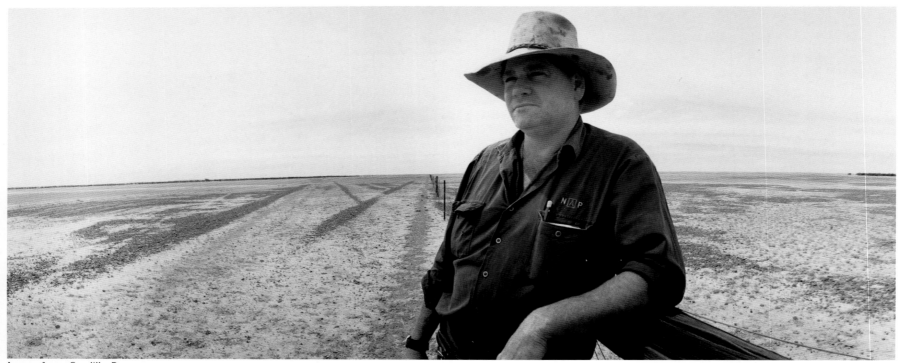

Lance from Cordillo Downs

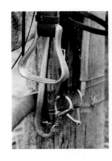

Contents

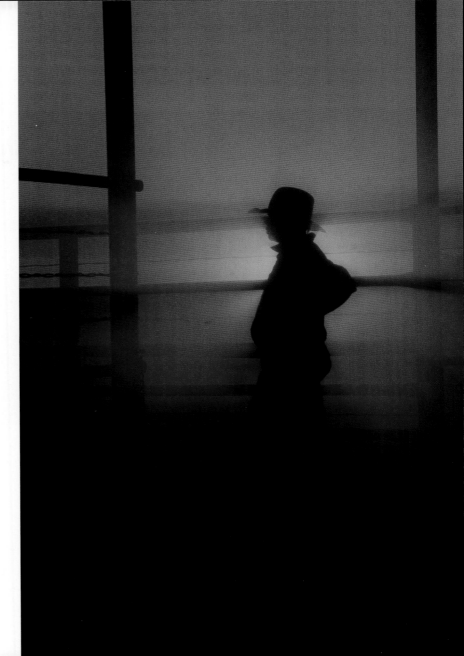

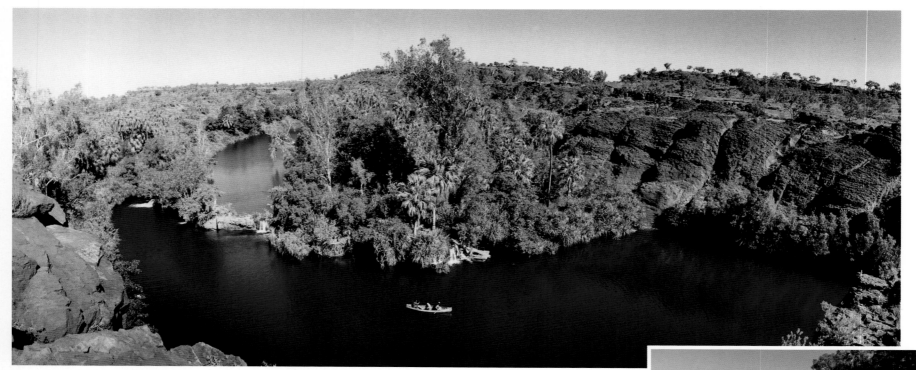

The spectacular Lawn Hill Gorge

A Note from the Photographer

Of all the areas I have travelled taking photographs, there is nowhere I enjoy more than the outback areas of Queensland, and I guess for this reason, it is where I get the best images.

Leesa helping me paddle through the Gorge

12

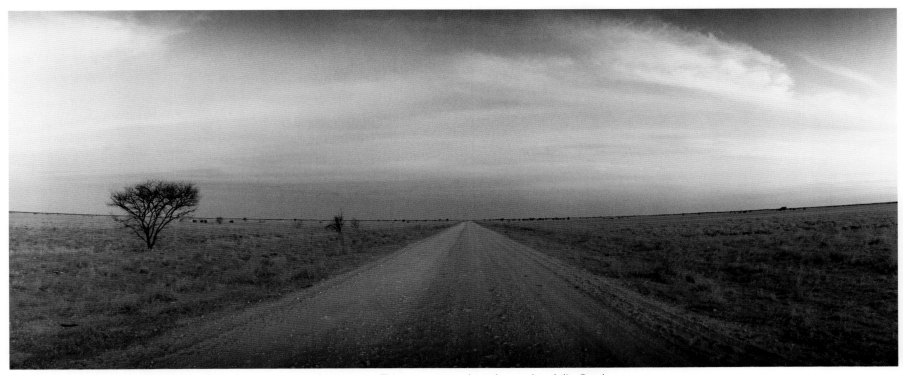

Early into our trip we experienced the first of many spectacular sunsets. This one occurred on the road to Julia Creek

So when I began the photography for this, my third book, it was the natural place to start. For one of these trips I was fortunate enough to be able to include my wife Suellen and two children, Leesa and Stephen. We initially travelled to Millungera Station, north of Julia Creek where I did several days of photography before continuing on to the Lawn Hill National Park. The gorge was spectacular and although it was mid-winter it was easy to lose ourselves for a day enjoying the water. We then continued on to Riversleigh where we enjoyed more water and viewed fossils and the "Grotto".

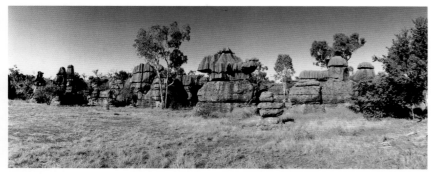
Limestone formations known as "The Grotto" near Riversleigh

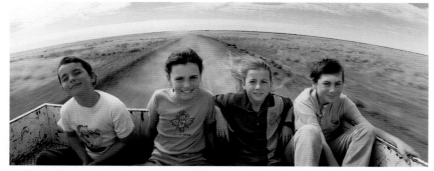
(L-R): Stephen, Leesa, Jade Roberts and Warwick Roberts travelling on Austral Downs

From here it was on to Austral Downs in the Northern Territory near Camoweal. Not only did Austral Downs provide the opportunity for some great photography, it provided a chance for the children to mix with some other children, Warwick and Jade Roberts.

We then travelled to Tobermorey Station, a property in the Northern Territory west of Urandangi and then down through Boulia to the Diamantina Lakes National Park. Our campsite was on the banks of the Diamantina River adjacent to a large permanent waterhole, the bird life was quite amazing.

The Diamantina Lakes National Park borders onto Davenport Downs, which was our next stop. The manager was Jack Morris. Jack was the head stockman in the camp at Nappa Merrie, which featured in my first book and was manager at Juanbung, which featured, in my second book. So naturally, it was only fitting that I should go to Jack when looking for images for book 3.

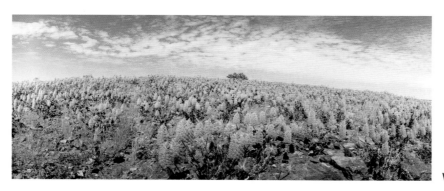
Wildflowers on Tobermorey Station

From here it was back home to Rockhampton. The trip had not only produced the photographic opportunities that I had hoped for, but proved to be one of our best times together as a family.

Several months later various opportunities arose which allowed me to take photographs on Moray Downs west of Clermont in Central Queensland and on Vanrook, north of Karumba in the Gulf.

It was late 2001 when we sold the last copies of my first book "A Taste of the Land", so I had to get my act together and finish the photography for "A Day in the Outback".

I felt I needed a few more images so I picked an area of the State I hadn't been to before, around Windorah and Birdsville.

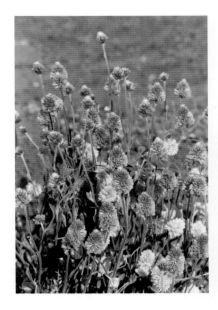

Wildflowers on
Tobermorey Station

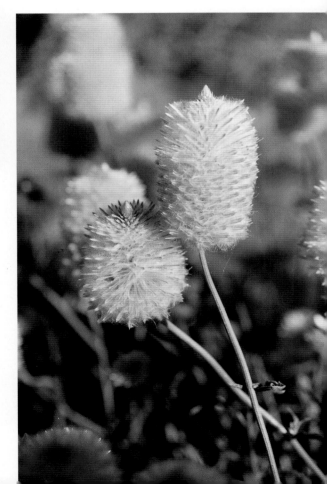

As this western country usually does, it provided some great images. The properties visited were Keeroongooloo south-east of Windorah, Durrie just east of Birdsville and Cordillo Downs in the north-east corner of South Australia. Of all the roads I have ever driven on, the track to Cordillo Downs would, without a doubt, be the worst, amazingly though I did not get a flat tyre.

In addition to all these new images, I have included what I consider to be the outstanding shots from "A Taste of the Land", my first book which has sold out and won't be reprinted.

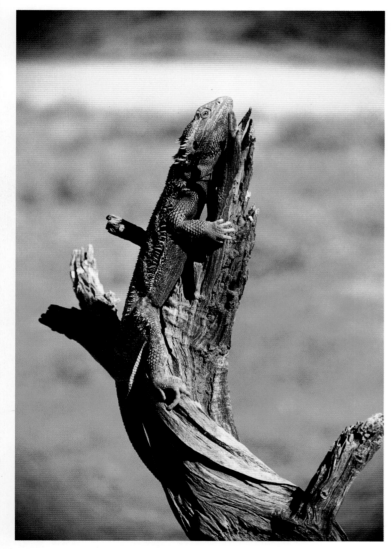

There are many people to thank for their assistance in the production of this book. They are too numerous to name, but to all of the wonderful people on the properties I visited, thank you very much. The hospitality of people in the Outback is always extraordinary. One of the great rewards of doing this kind of photography is the wonderful people that I meet, and to them all, thank you very much.

Thanks once again to John for his expertise in developing and printing the images.

Finally, and most importantly, thank you Suellen for all your help and support.

Mark Coombe

Mark Coombe
Rockhampton
2002

One of the many lizards near the road between Boulia and the Diamantina Lakes National Parks

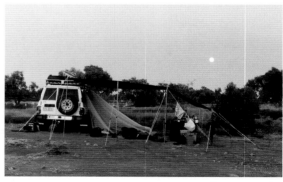

Facing page: A full moon sinks in the west as the sun rises over Diamantina Lakes.

Our camp site

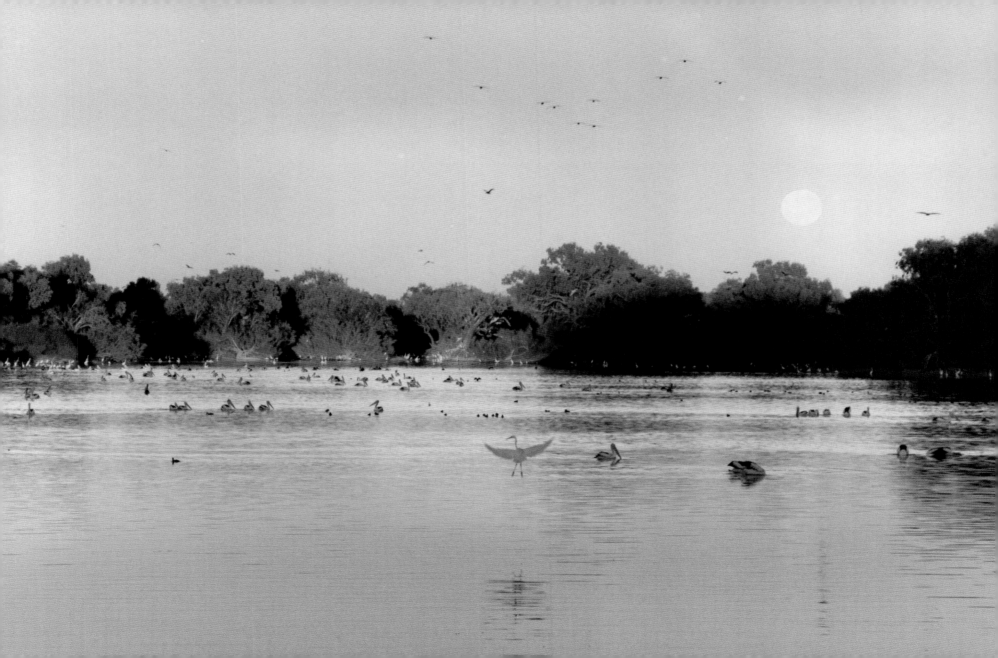

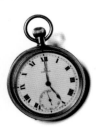

DAWN

A time of day that signifies a hive of activity in preparation for the day ahead. Catching horses, preparing equipment, it's a chance to get as much done as possible before the day heats up. It's the coolest part of the day and from my experience, without a doubt, the most spectacular.

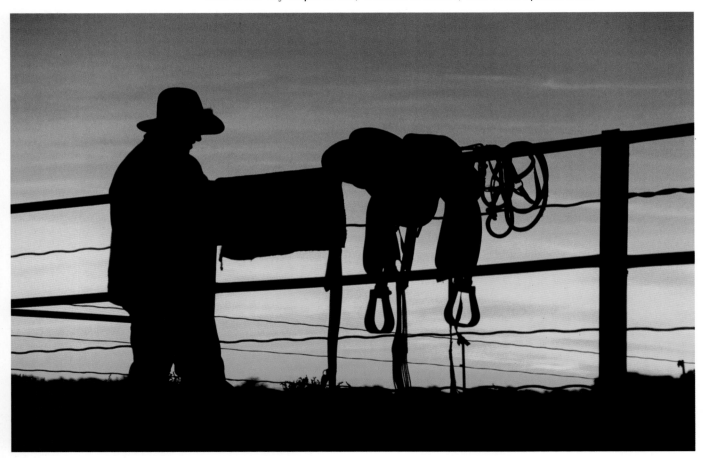

Getting saddle equipment ready at Davenport Downs before catching the horses. Once caught and saddled the horses are trucked out to an appropriate place in the paddock where the muster begins. The long distances are covered by motorbikes and helicopters

Facing page: Running in the horses at Nappa Merrie

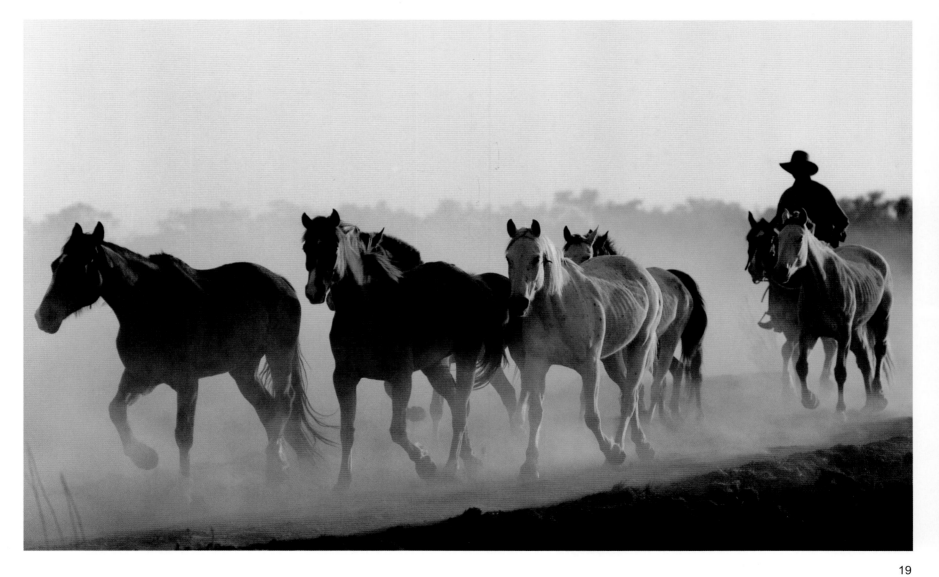

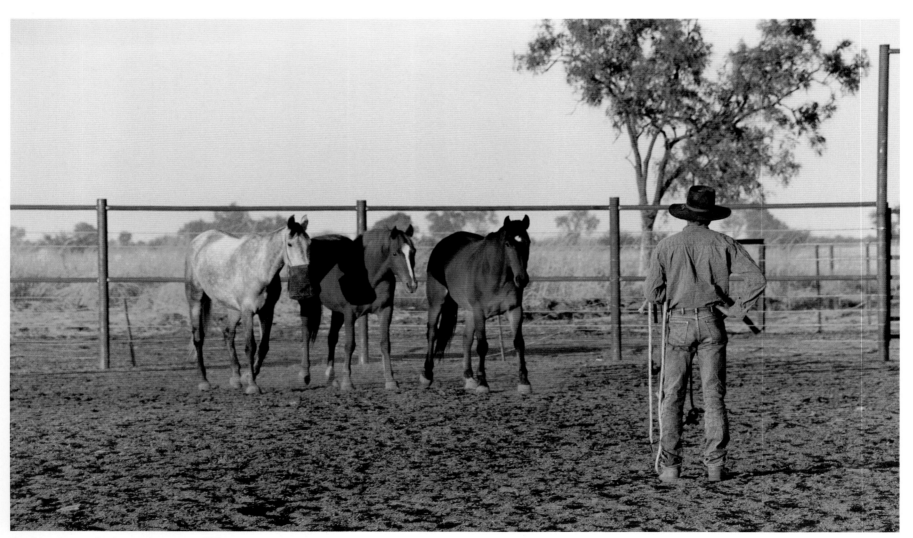

Catching horses in the stock camp at Millungera

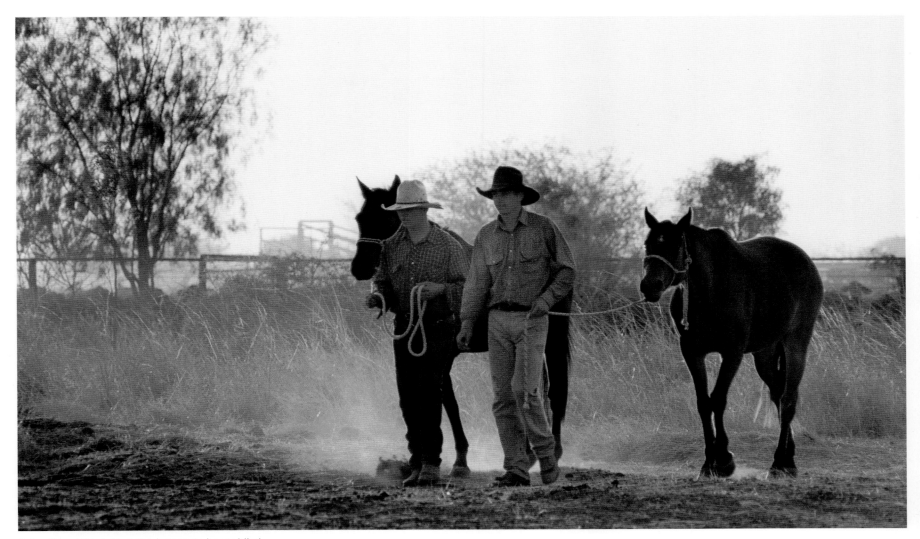

A familiar sight, taking the horses to be saddled

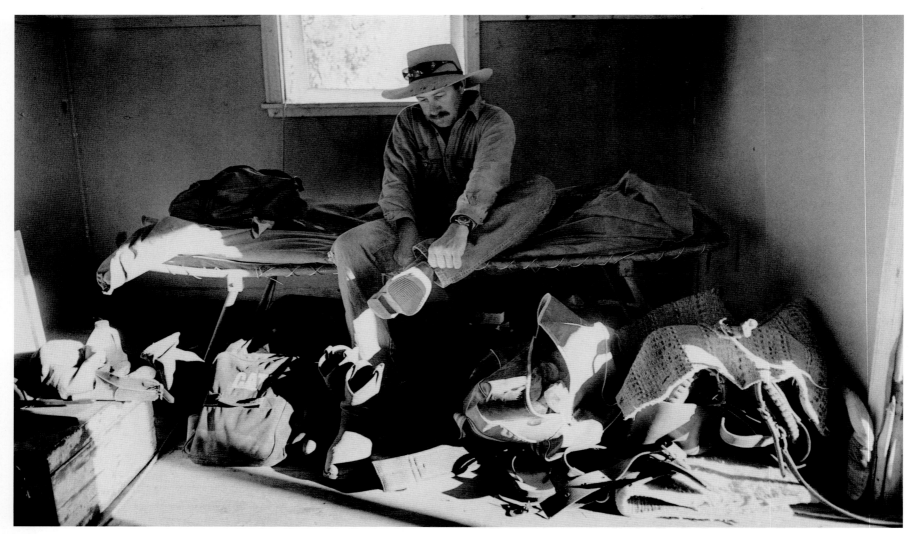

Selecting the right boots for the day

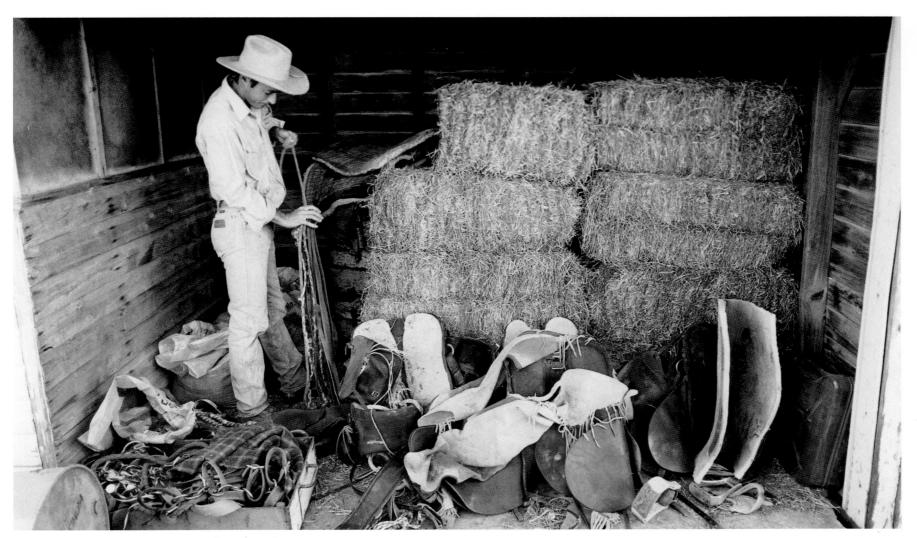

Getting gear ready in the stockcamp at Keeroongooloo

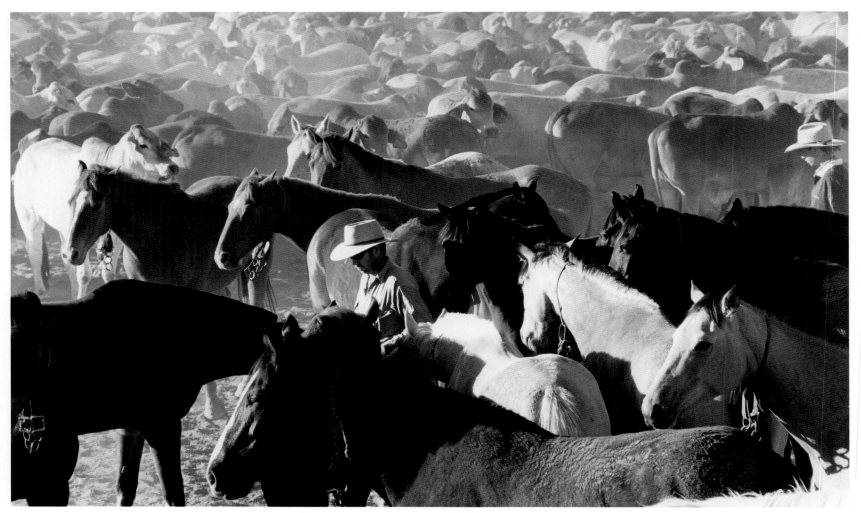

Catching horses in the stockcamp at Keeroongooloo. As with many stock camps, the horses are kept in the same overnight yards as the cattle and are moved with them during the day to the next camp. This enables fresh horses to be available each day

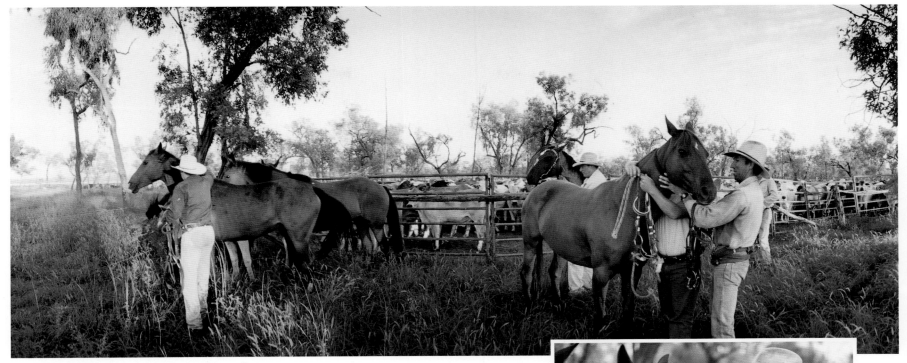

Getting prepared for the day ahead at Moray Downs

Rusty Prentice, a well known figure in Central
Queensland and manager of Moray Downs,
catching his horse for the day

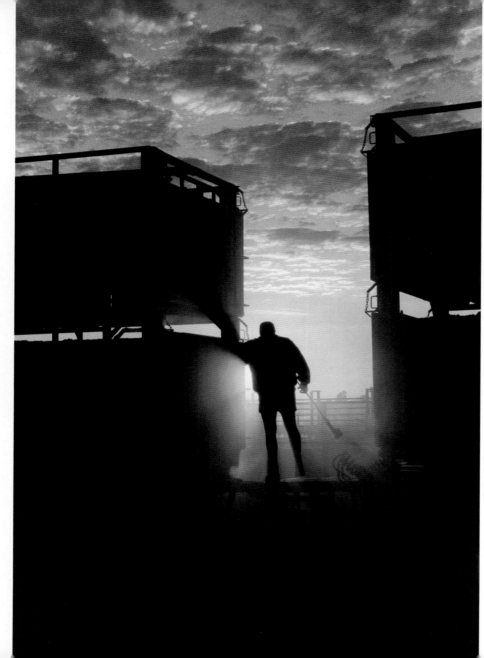

Road Trains of Australia is a livestock carrying business based in Darwin in the Northern Territory. Each year the company moves around 20 000 decks of cattle, at an average of 28 head per deck, that's around 560 000 cattle. They carry cattle all over Queensland, the Northern Territory and the Kimberly Region of Western Australia. Their 38 prime movers average around 150 000km each per year.

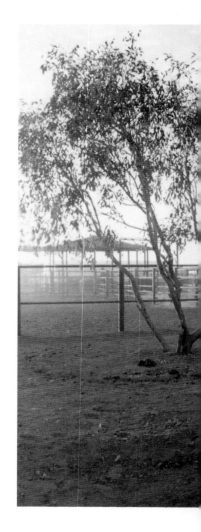

Like the stockmen and women, the truckies that drive the road trains are up early loading cattle

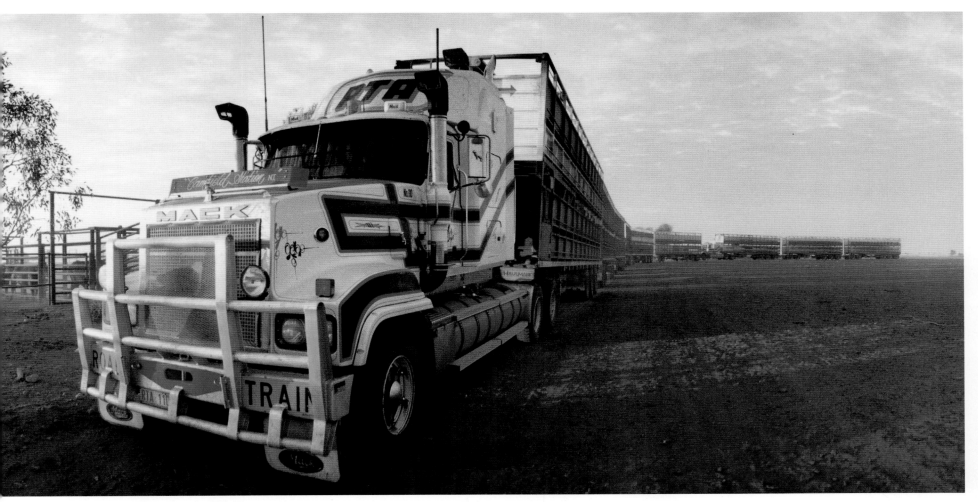

Loading young cattle at Austral Downs for their transfer to another of the A.A. Company properties.

Over leaf: Loading the decks

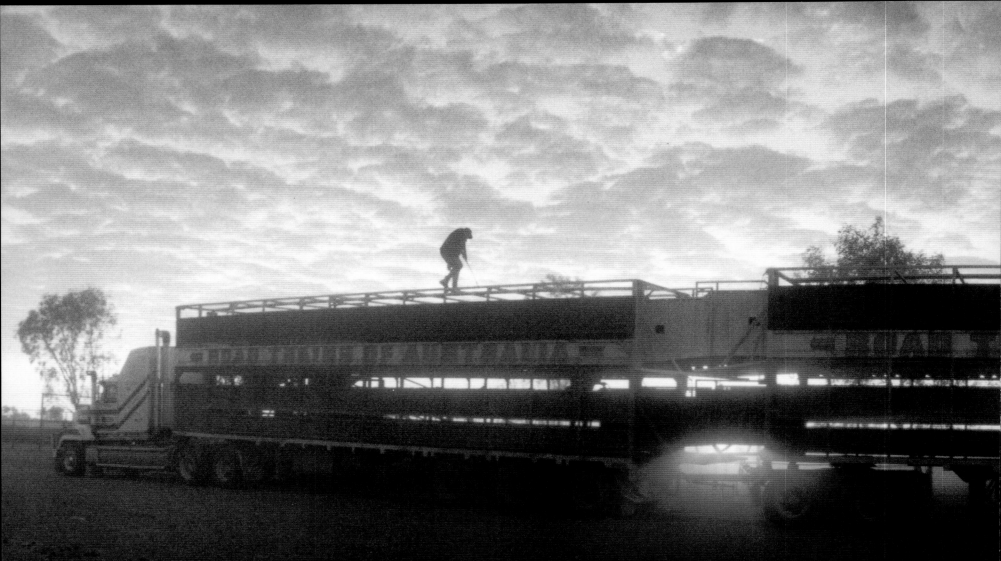

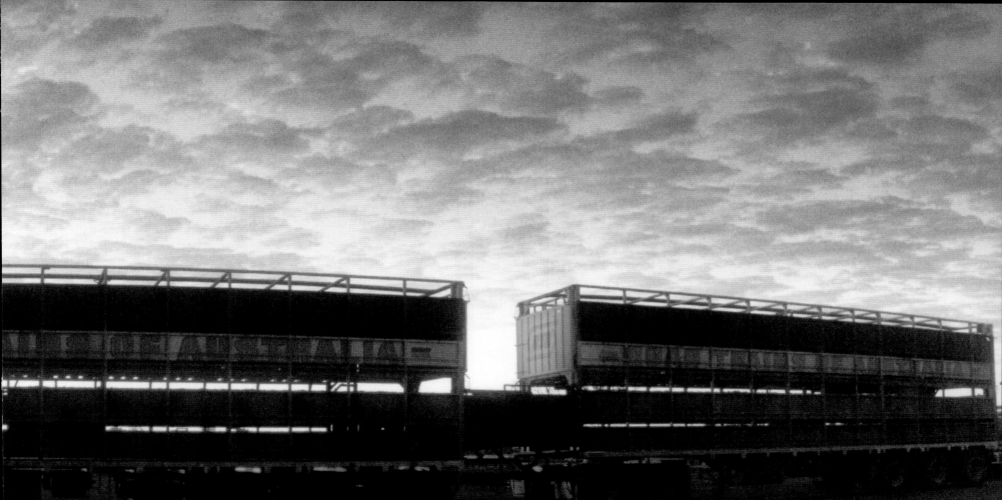

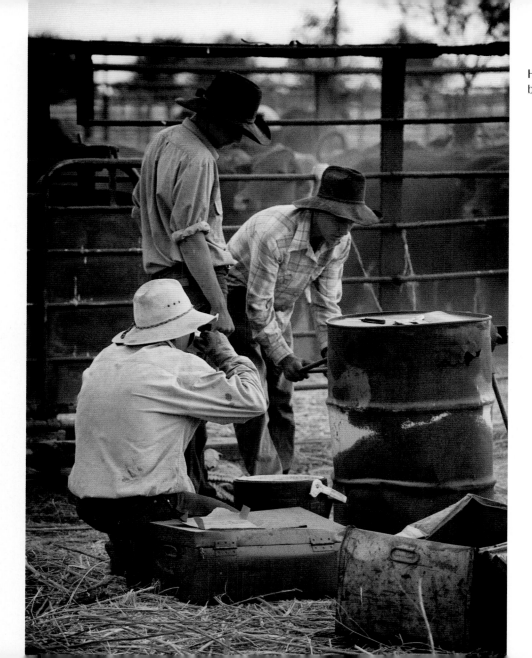

Having a drink and heating up the
branding irons

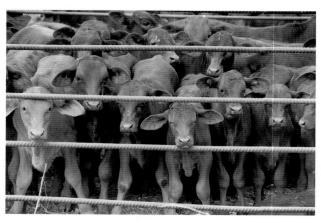

Waiting their turn for the branding iron

Facing page: Yarding up

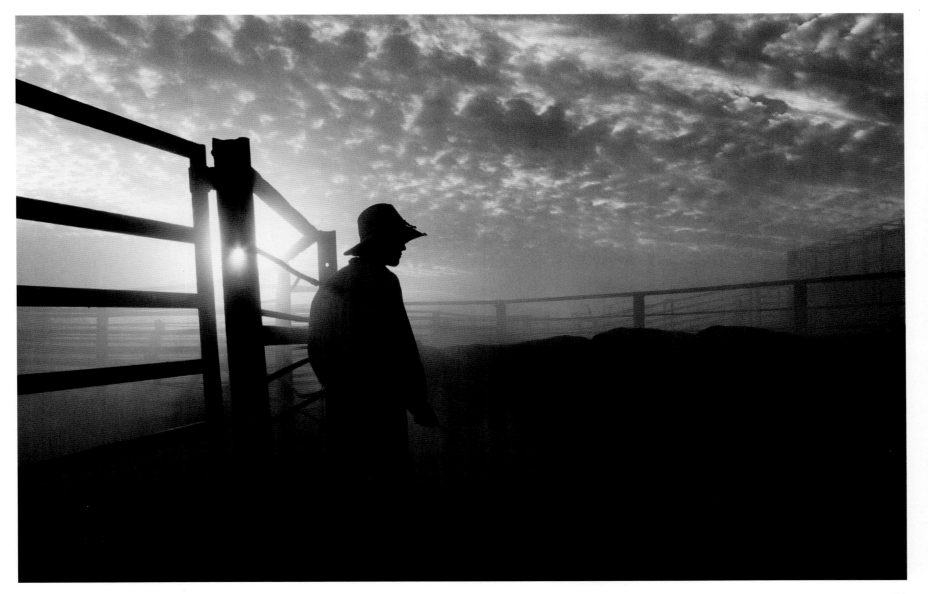

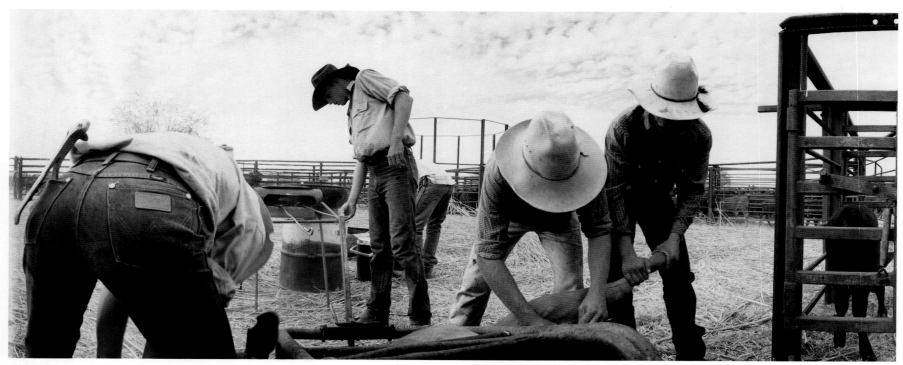

All hands on deck

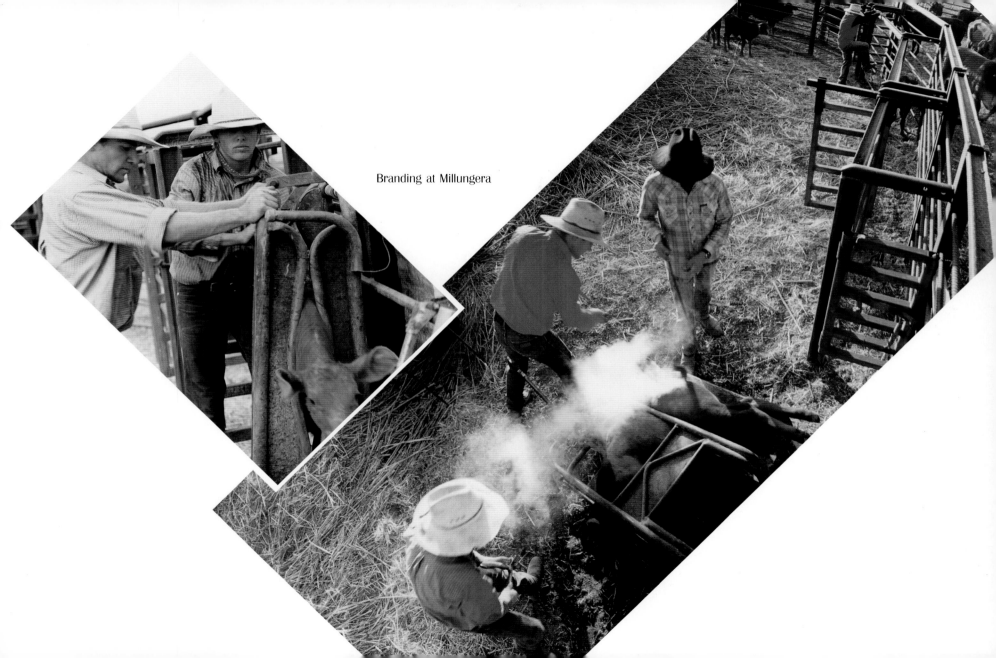

Branding at Millungera

Dawn at Cordillo Downs

Cordillo Downs was taken over by Peter Waite in 1883 to become one of a string of properties owned by the Beltona Pastoral Company. It was stocked initially with 10 312 sheep, 580 cattle, 28 horses and 1 camel.

The buildings at Cordillo have curved roofing, this came about because of the lack of timber in the area for beams. Curved iron was easy to transport by camel and once riveted together was self-supporting.

In 1888, 82 000 sheep were shorn in the 128 stand shed by hand shears.

In 1907, mechanical shearing was introduced and the Federal Sheep Shearing Company had the contract to shear 36 000 sheep. They had 42 men (30 shearers) and took 3 weeks to complete the task with the record tally of 187 sheep for one man in one day.

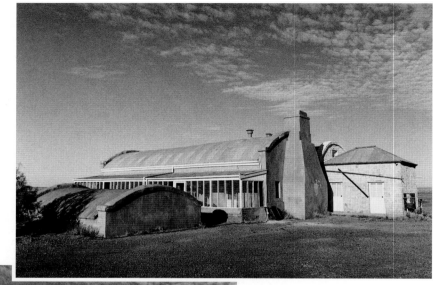

Buildings at Cordillo Downs

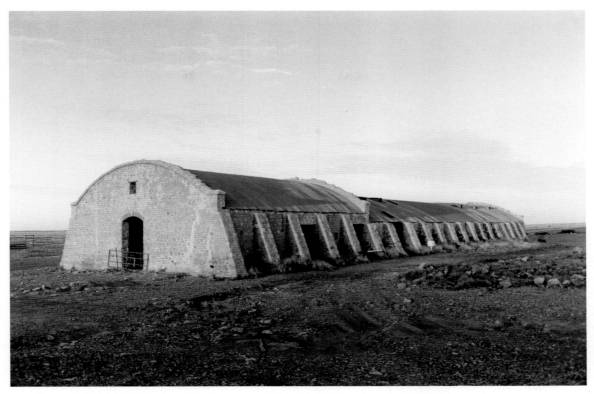

Cordillo Downs shearing shed

In 1941 dingoes killed most of the lamb drop, and as a result the sheep were removed and it became a cattle station.

Cordillo Downs was purchased by the Brook family in 1981.

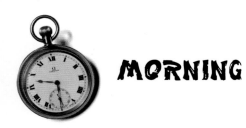

MORNING

By mid-morning work is in full swing, if its mustering, cattle are starting to come together or being moved from one camp to the next. Yard work is well underway and the temperature is on the rise.

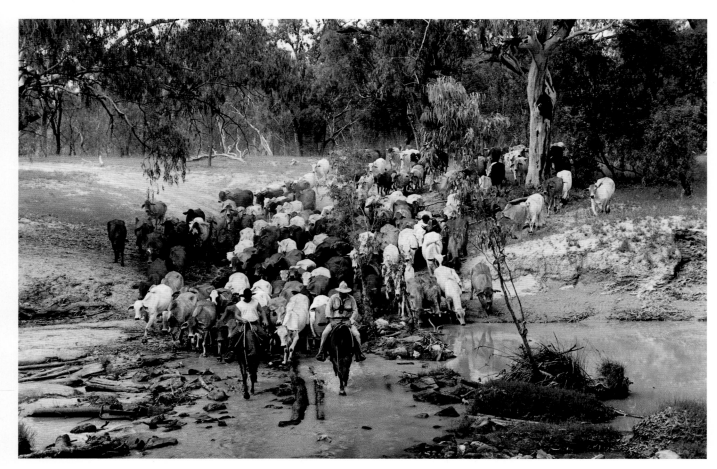

Leading cattle through the
Carmichael Creek

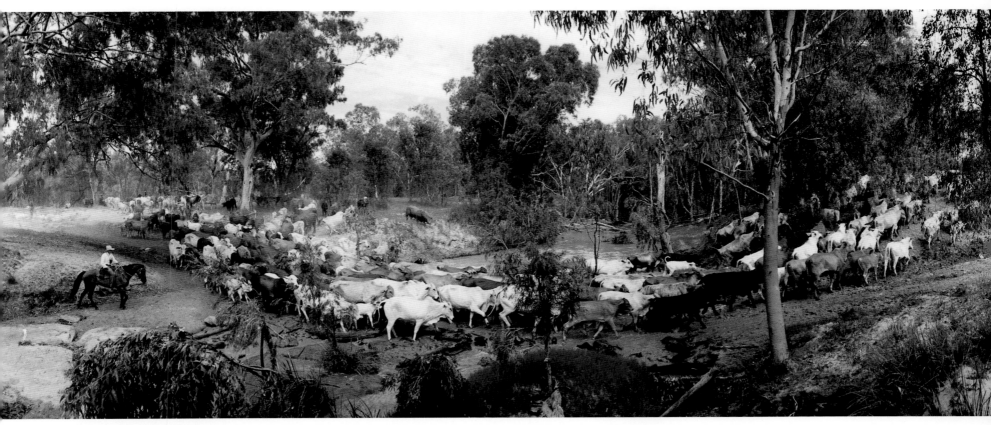

Crossing the Carmichael

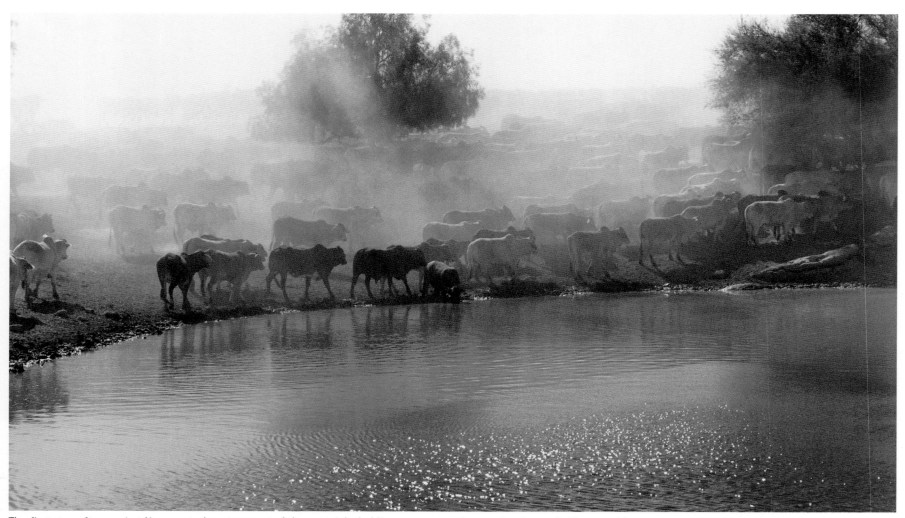

The first stop after moving Keeroongooloo steers out of the overnight holding pen was at the nearby ring tank. They would not see water again until late in the day when stopping at the next camp

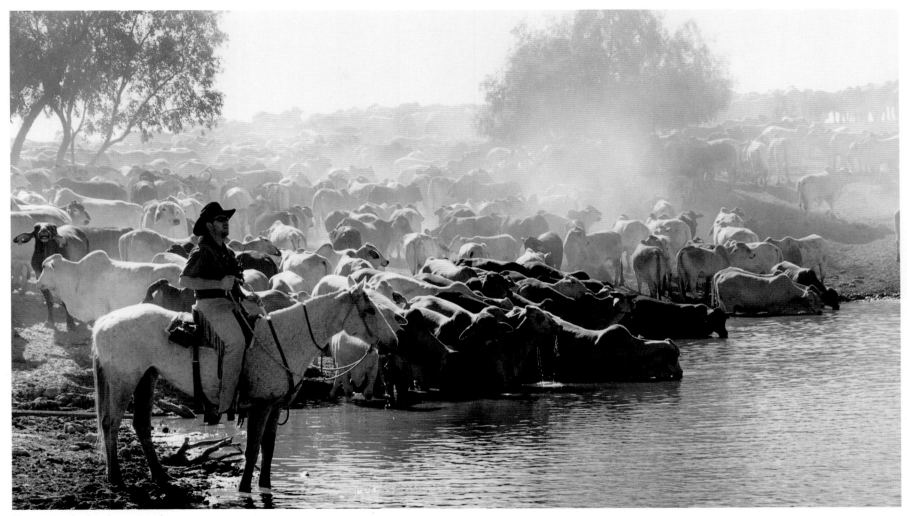

Horses too had to be watered

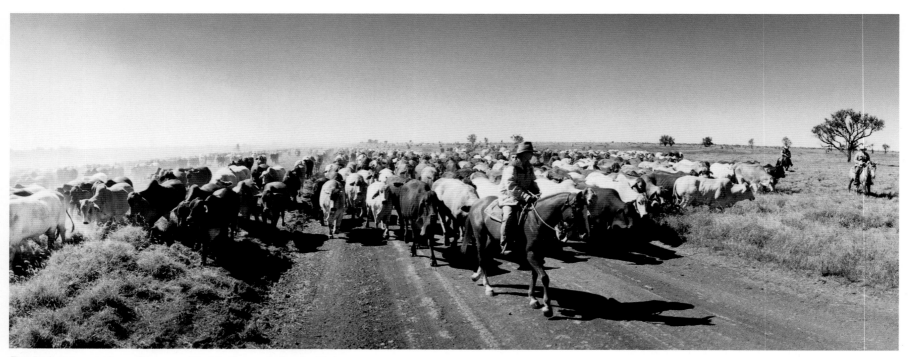

Finished steers at Moray Downs walking to the yards for drafting

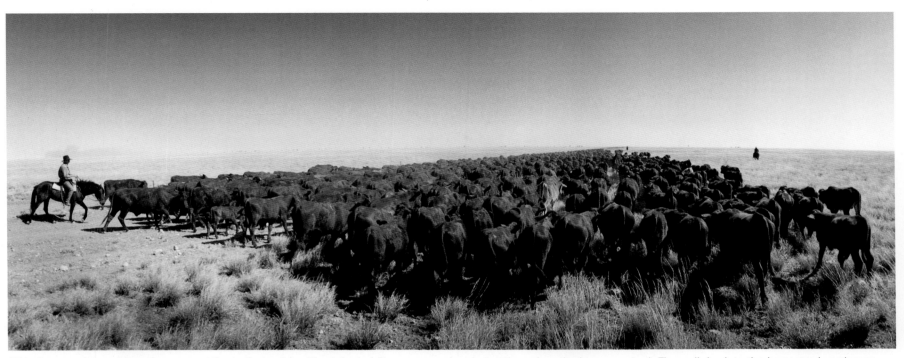

With the use of motorbikes these young Santa Gertrudis cattle at Austral Downs were already together when the horses arrived. The walk back to the homestead yards was well underway by mid-morning

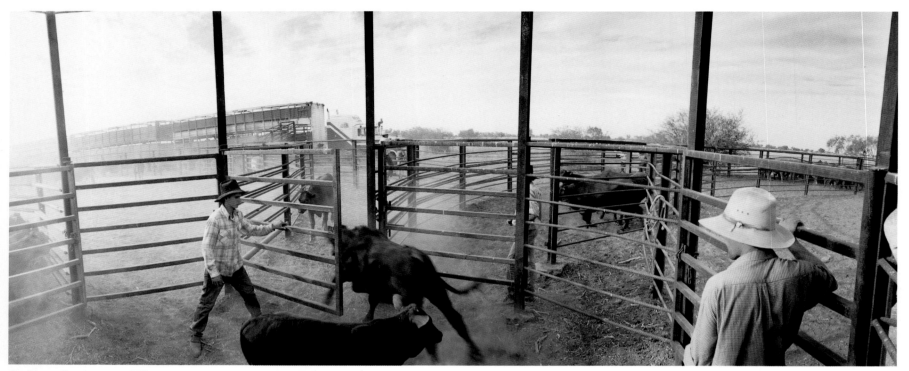

Drafting off weaners at Millungera

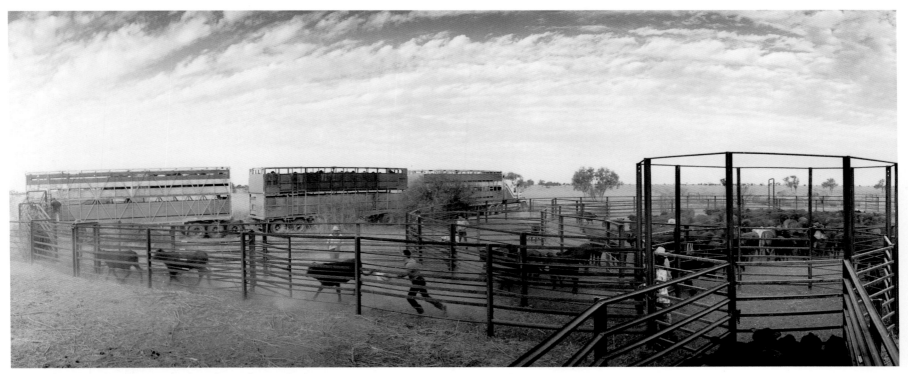

and loading them for transport back to the station yards

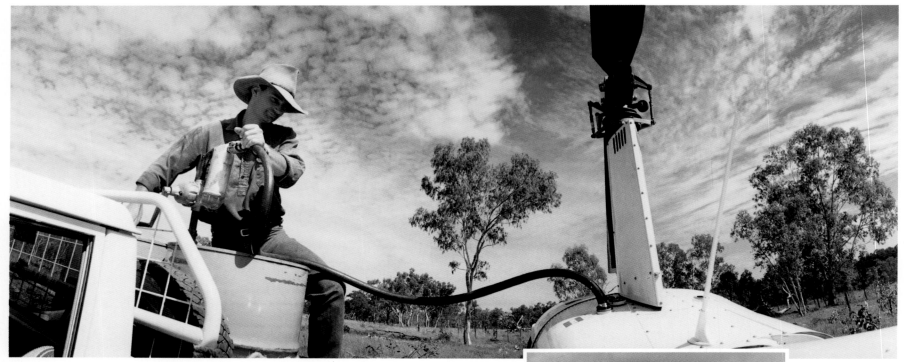

Helicopter, Kilo Kilo Gulf, being filled with fuel by Rob Pegg at Moray Downs.

With a range of about 3 hours fifteen minutes, the Robinson 22 is one of the most common helicopters used for mustering throughout Australia. This helicopter is operated by Webb Helicopters, a company based in Emerald which covers the entire state of Queensland. They have 9 Robinson 22 helicopters and the 10 pilots with the company average 700 – 900 hours flying time per year.

Kilo Kilo Gulf
pushing the mob

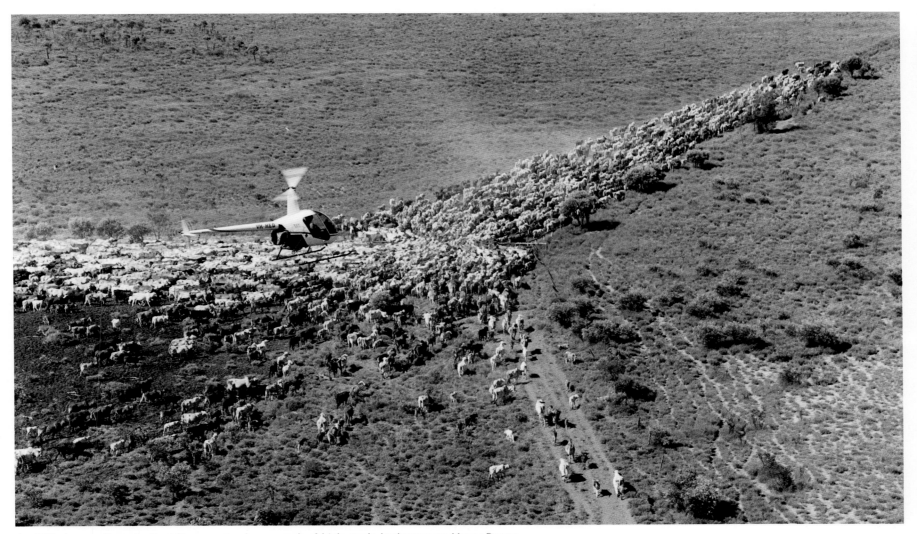

An R22 chopper flown by Kent Hansen sits above a mob of high grade brahmans on Moray Downs

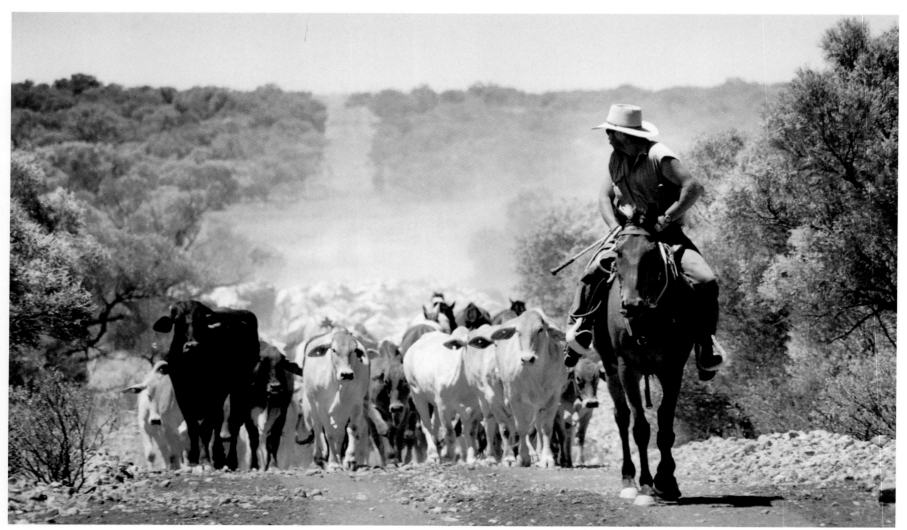

As the morning progressed, the mob being mustered at Keeroongooloo steadily grew

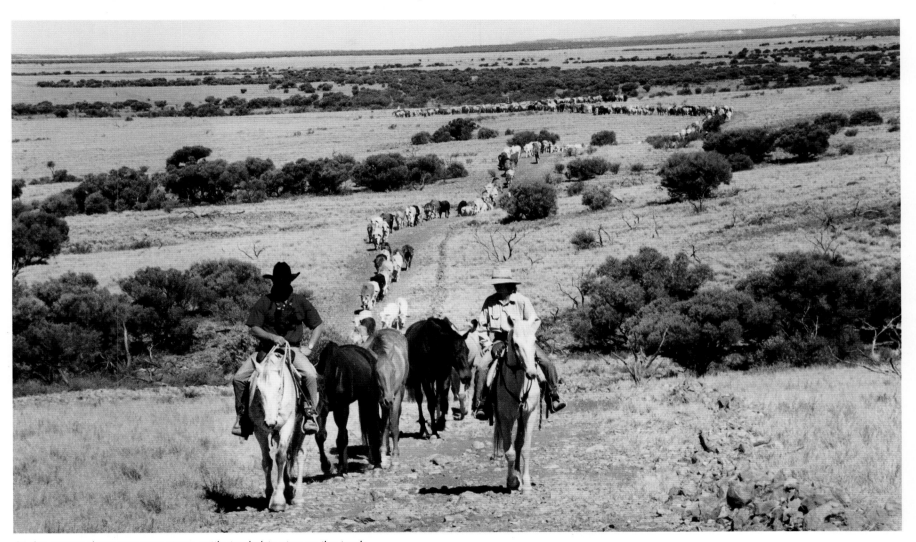

As the country here was very stony, cattle tended to stay on the track

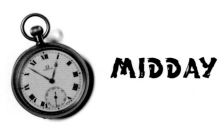

MIDDAY

The hottest time of the day. It's a chance to grab some lunch, often carried in saddle bags or in a vehicle nearby while the cattle are pulled up for a rest. For those working cattle in the yards they can normally boil the billy and grab a rest for an hour, if they're lucky.

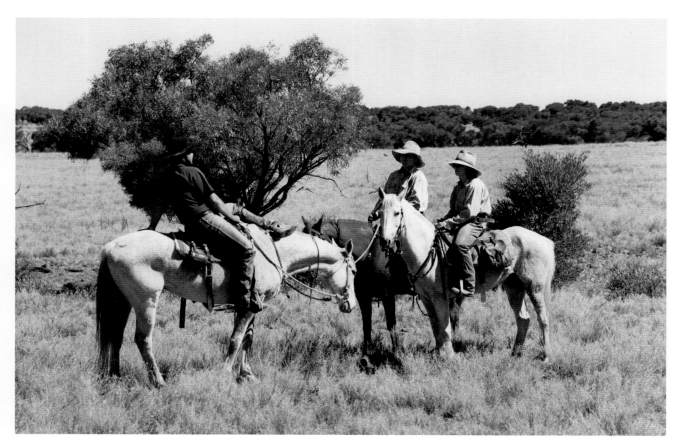

Resting near the mob

48

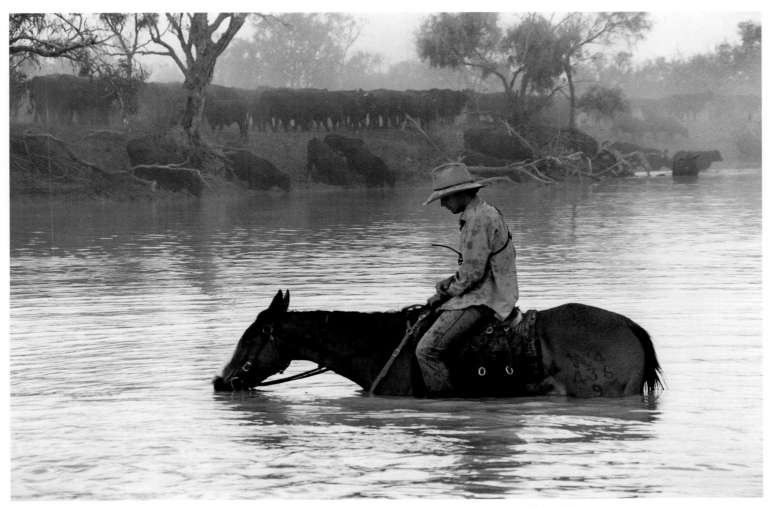

Time for a drink as a mob of Santa Gertrudis steers rest on a channel of the Cooper Creek at Nappa Merrie Station

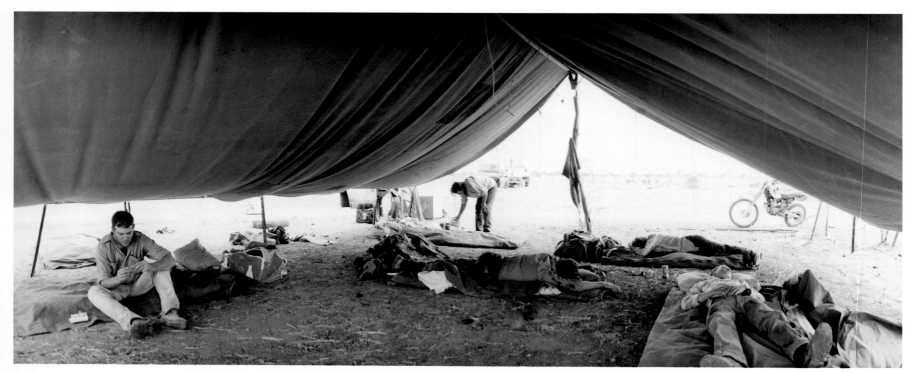

A chance to rest ...

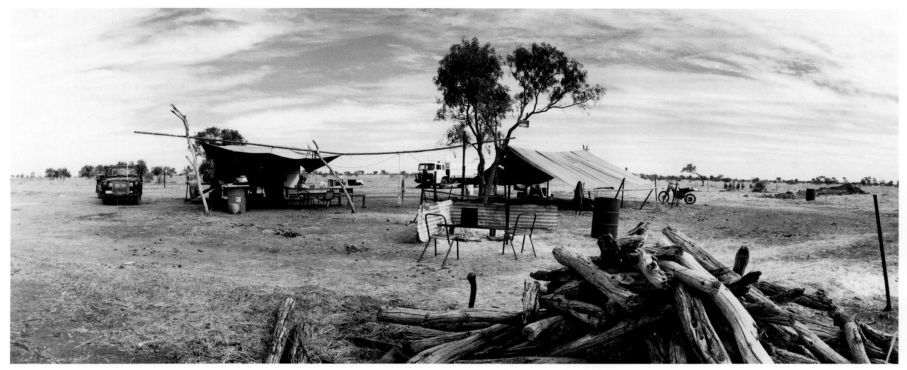

... in the Millungera stock camp

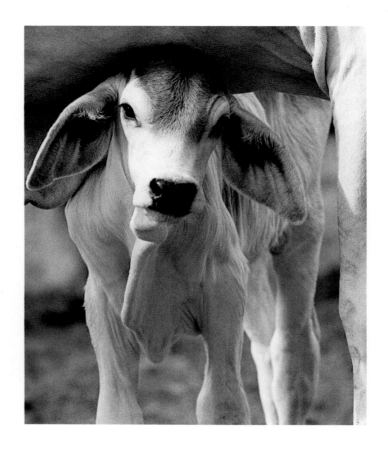

A young brahman calf rests in the safety beneath its' mother

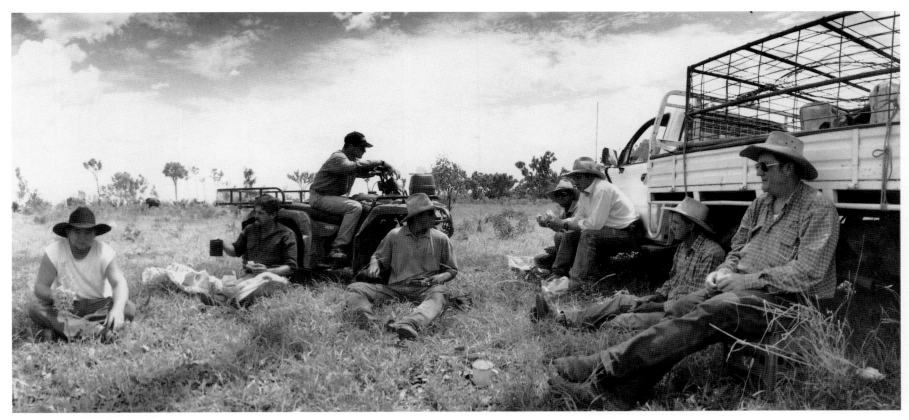

Lunch break at Moray Downs

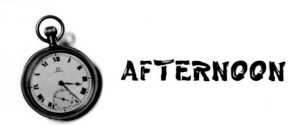

AFTERNOON

A time when the actual muster may be over and it's time to drive cattle to holding pens or yards. Often many kilometres have to be covered before darkness falls. If it's yard work then it's usually a rush to get all the cattle processed before days end.

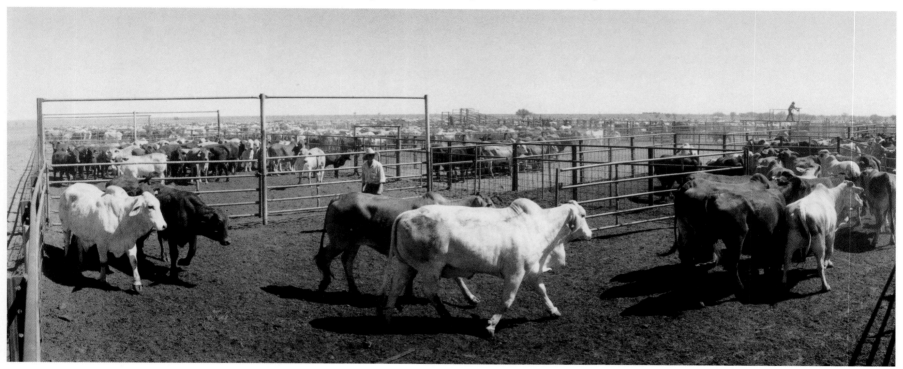

Working cattle at Keeroongooloo

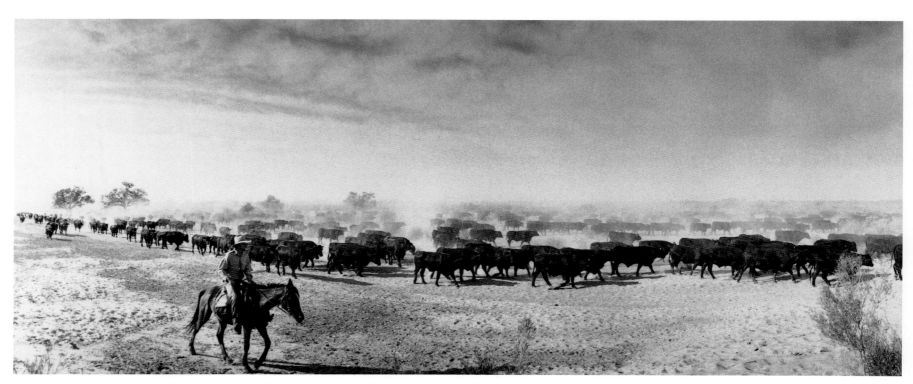
Moving around the sand dunes on Nappa Merrie Station

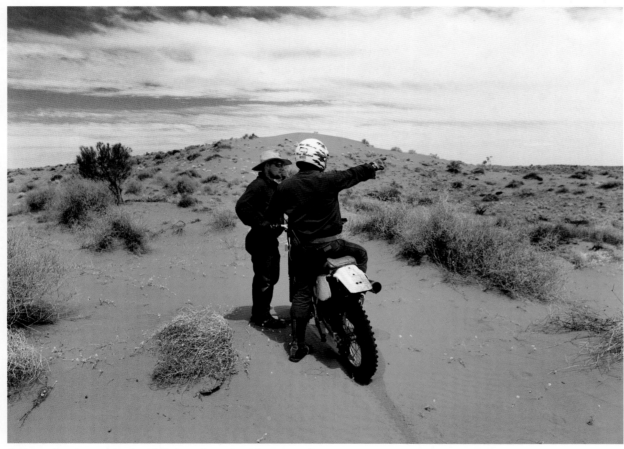

The excellent producing ability of this country and lack of pests has seen the Brook family producing organic beef off Cordillo Downs and their other stations in the West. Their beef is marketed under the brand name OBE Beef. Despite being on the edge of the Strezlecki Desert and the apparent lack of what would appear to be any decent feed, the Poll Hereford cattle were in superb condition.

Anthony Brooks and Lance Melksham from Cordillo Downs discuss the easiest way over the sand dunes

Facing page & over leaf: Crossing the dunes on Cordillo Downs

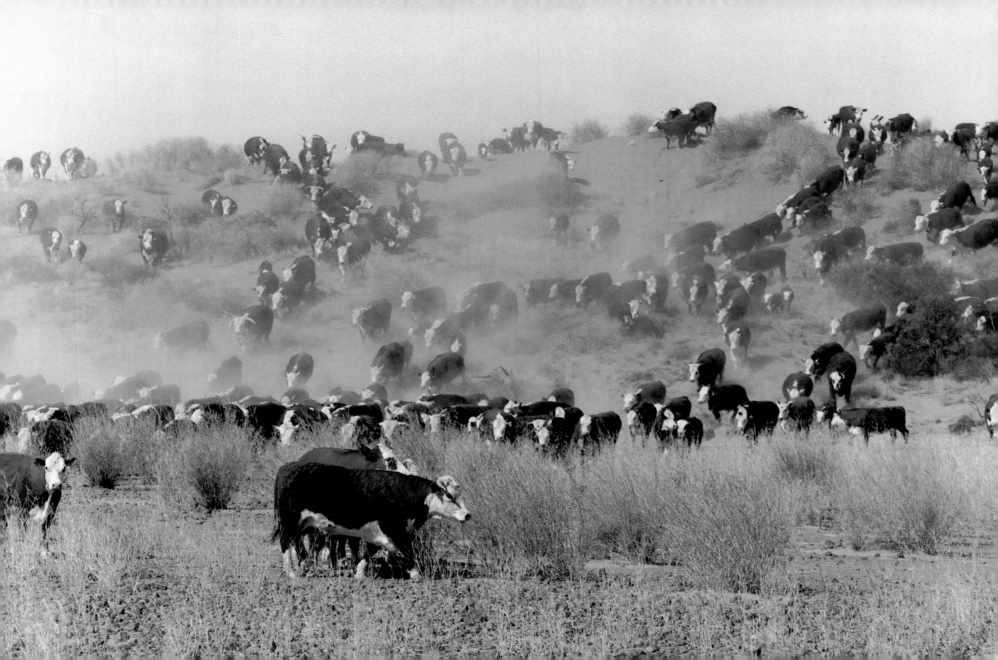

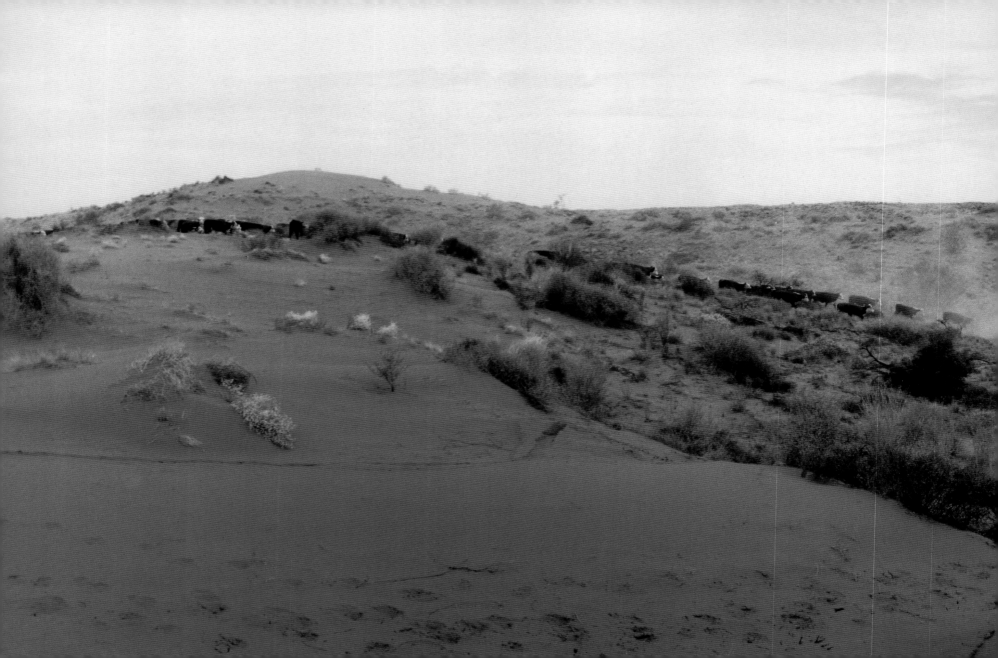

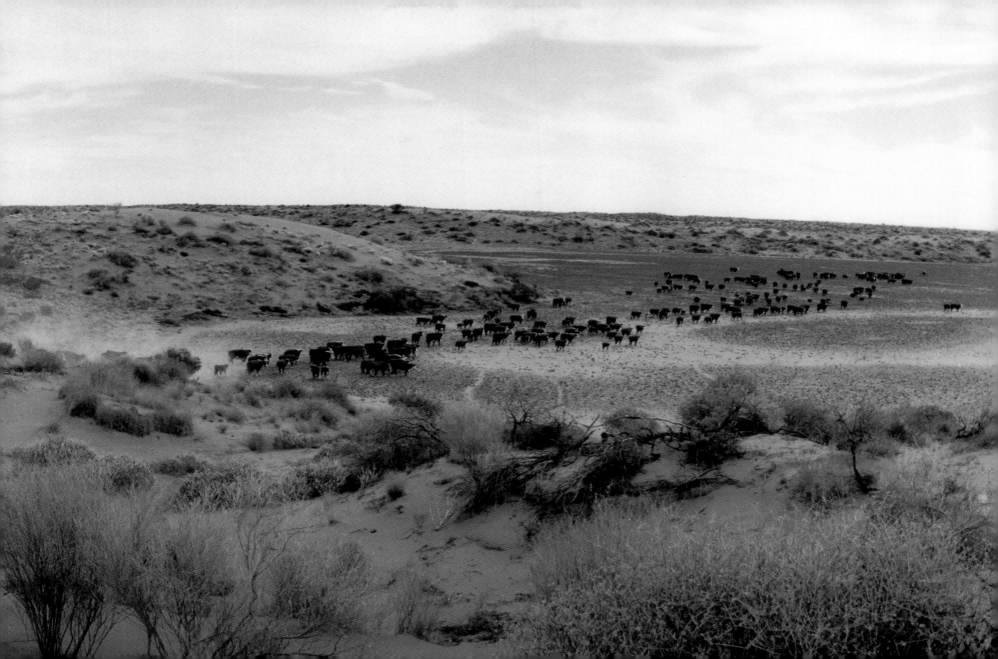

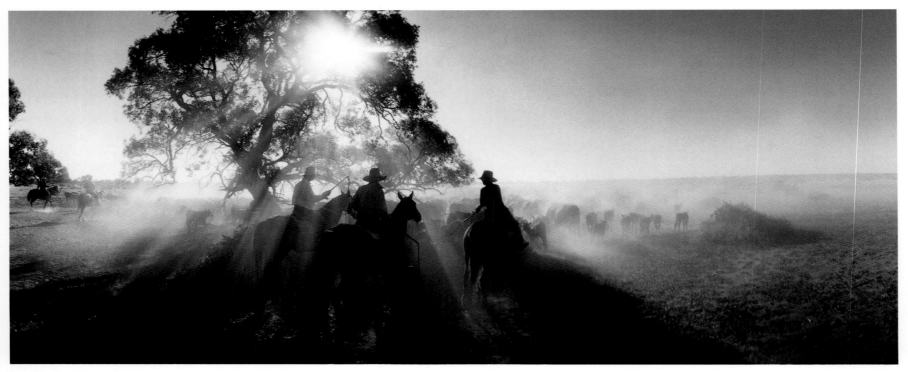

Dust on the tail

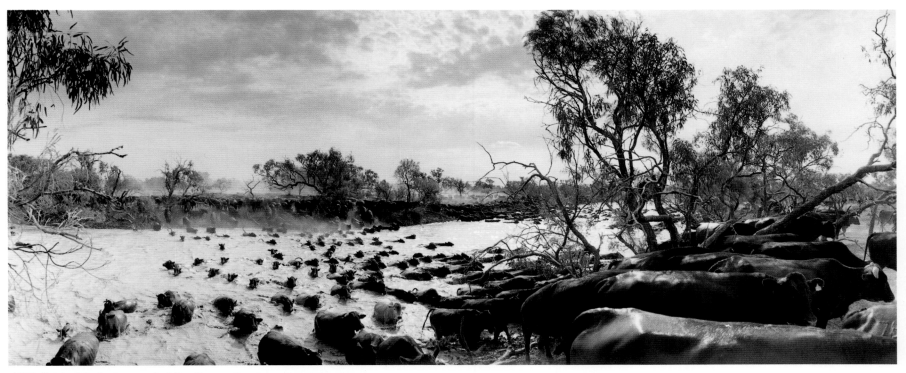

4000 finished bullocks crossing the Cooper Creek on Nappa Merrie

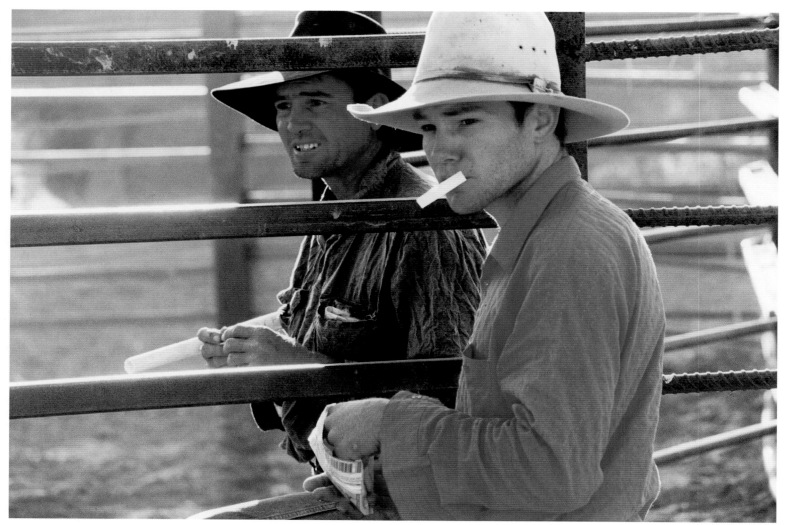

Time for a smoke

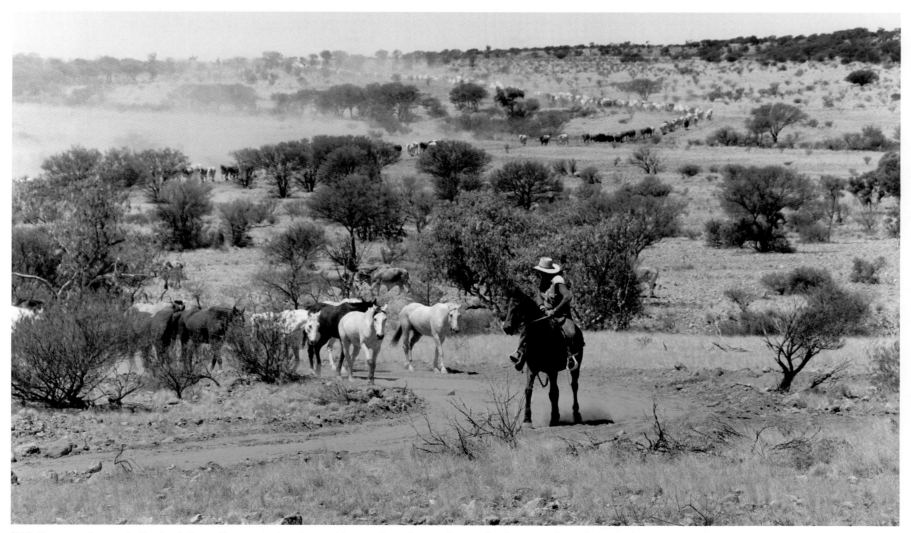

With the camp horses in the lead, these Keeroongooloo steers string out for miles as they snake their way through the rocky country to the yards

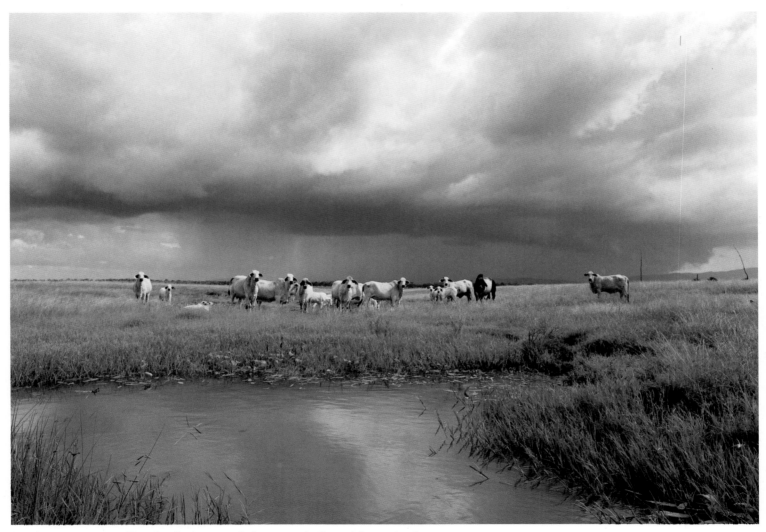

An afternoon storm at Waverley Station near St Lawrence in Central Queensland

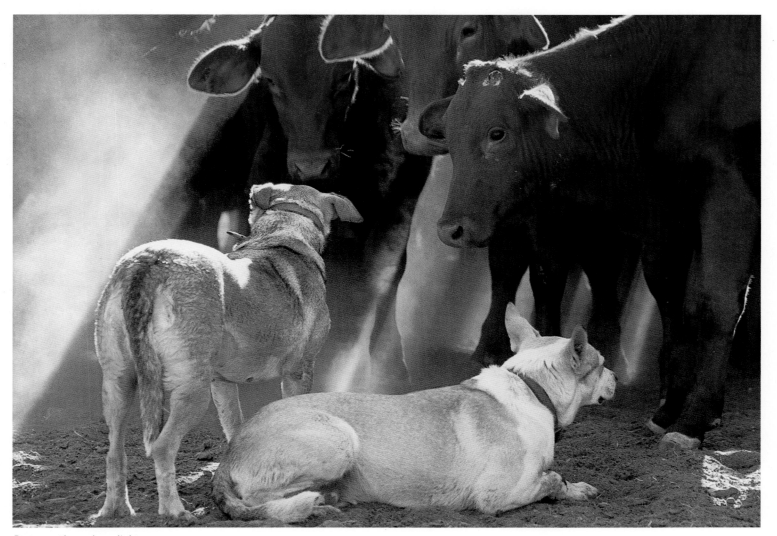

Dogs, cattle and sunlight

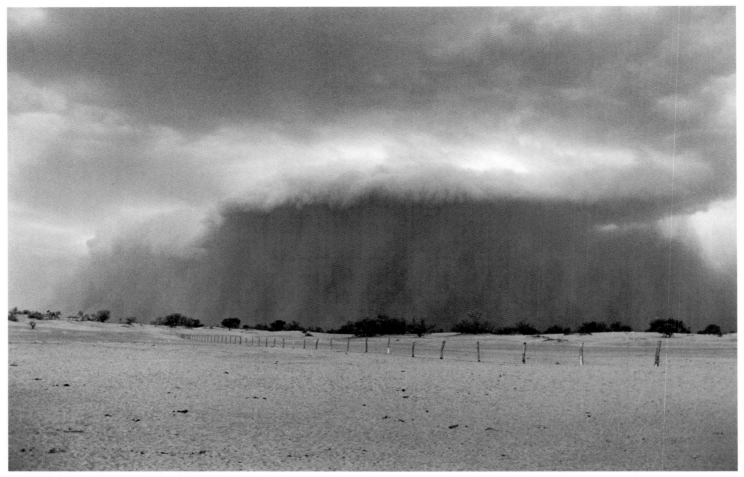

Dust storm at Barioolah on Nappa Merrie Station

This dust storm was formed by a micro-burst of strong winds forming ahead of an advancing line of thunderstorms associated with a frontal system.

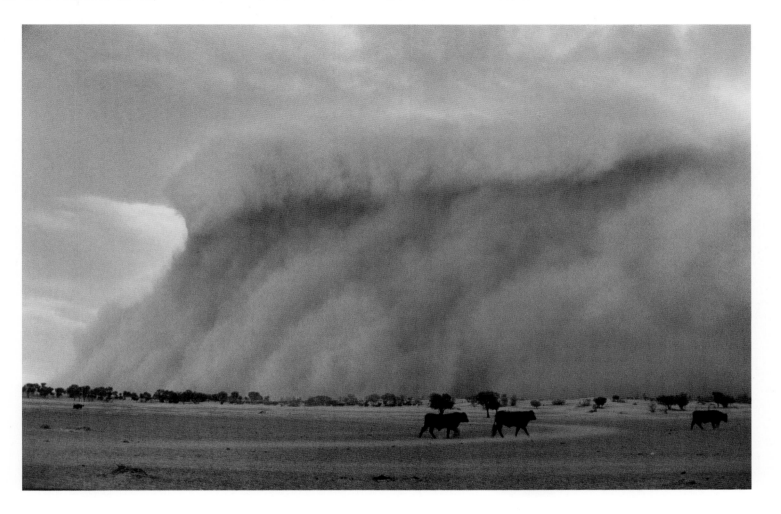

Strong winds, a very unstable atmosphere and hot dusty ground conditions combined to raise and swirl the dust through a considerable amount of the atmosphere and reduce visibility to a few metres. These dust storms associated with fronts and thunderstorms can extend for hundreds of kilometres in parts of inland Australia during the summer months.

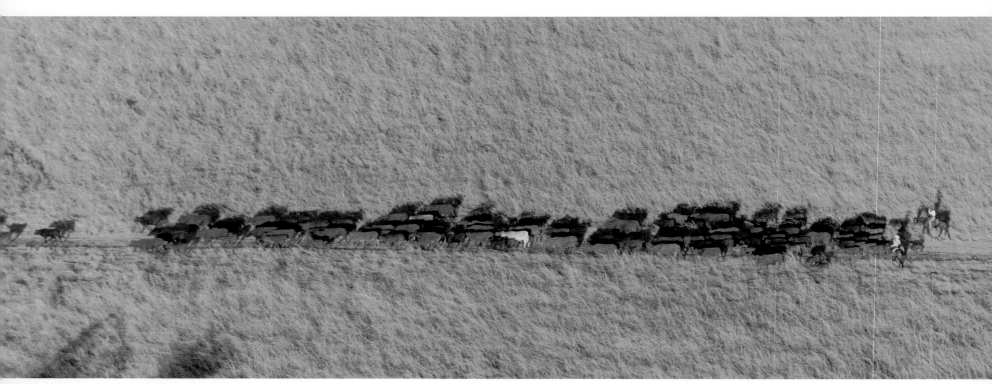

Santa Gertrudis breeders moving across the open country on Millungera

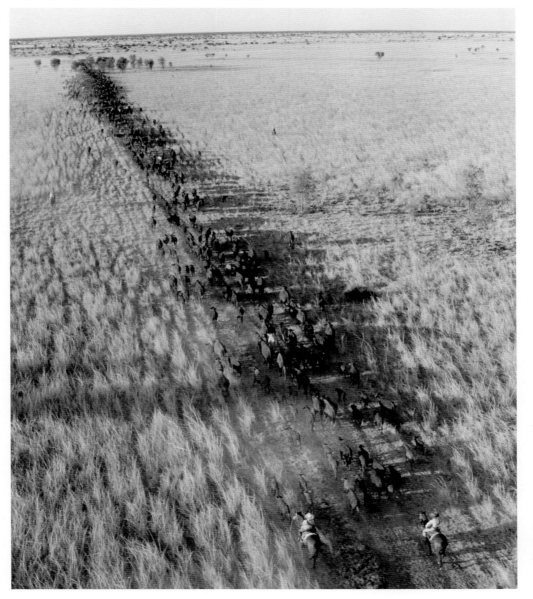

Cattle string out for miles as they make their way to the yards before nightfall

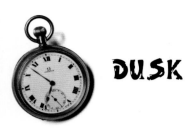

DUSK

Like the dawn, this is one of the most spectacular times in the Outback. The air starts to cool and the setting sun brings about the amazing colours for which the Australian Outback is renown. It is also a time for finishing yard work and getting mustered mobs into secure enclosures for the night.

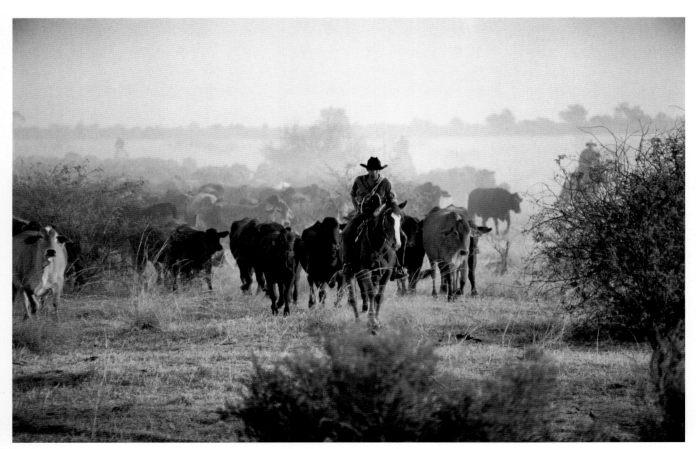

Leading the mob to the yards late in the day on Millungera

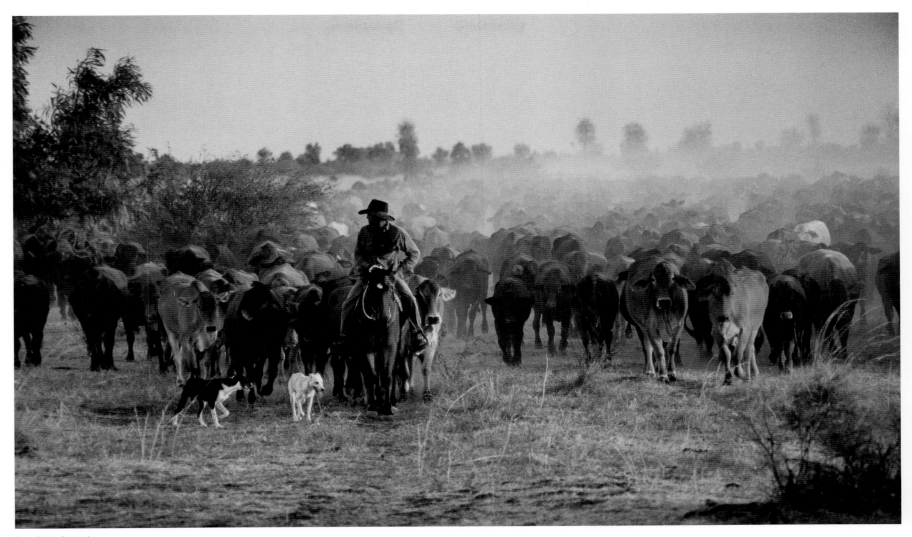

Leading them in

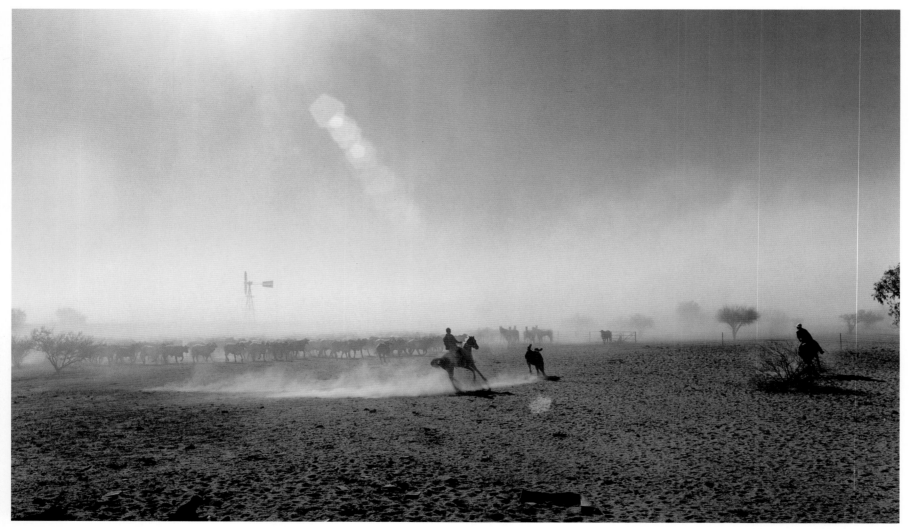

Yarding up at Kerroongooloo

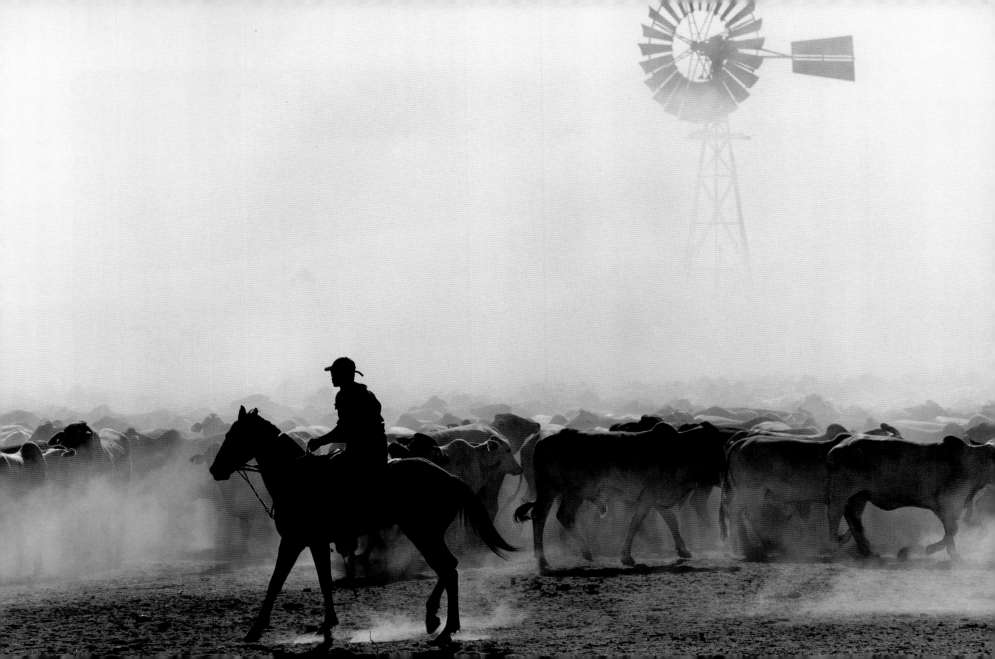

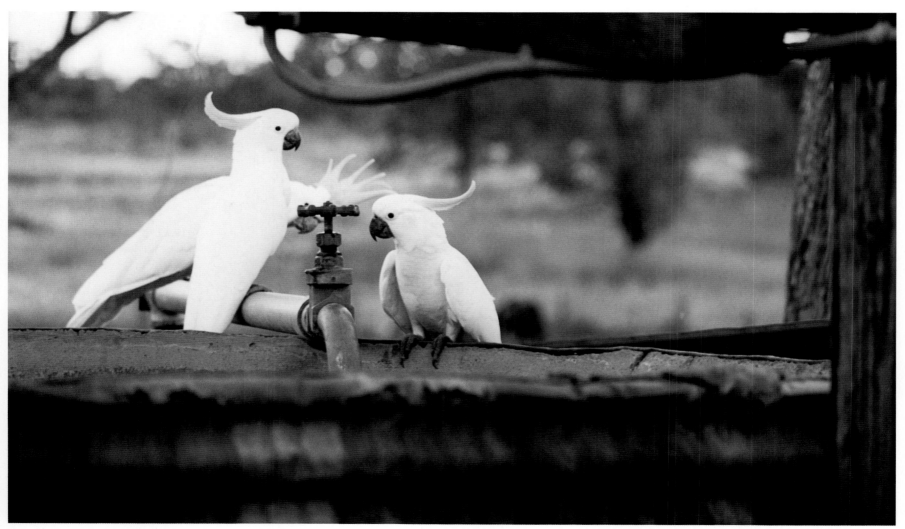

Cockatoos in for a late afternoon drink

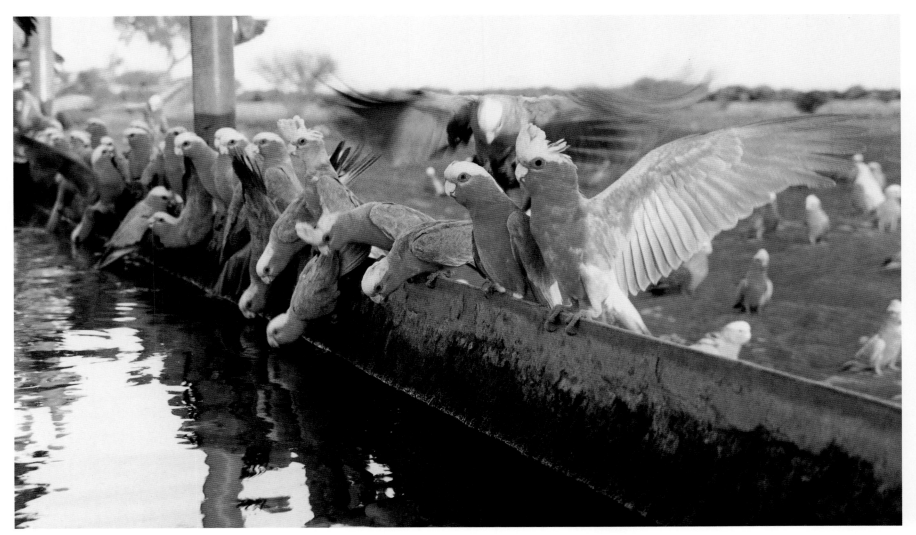

Galahs gathering at the trough

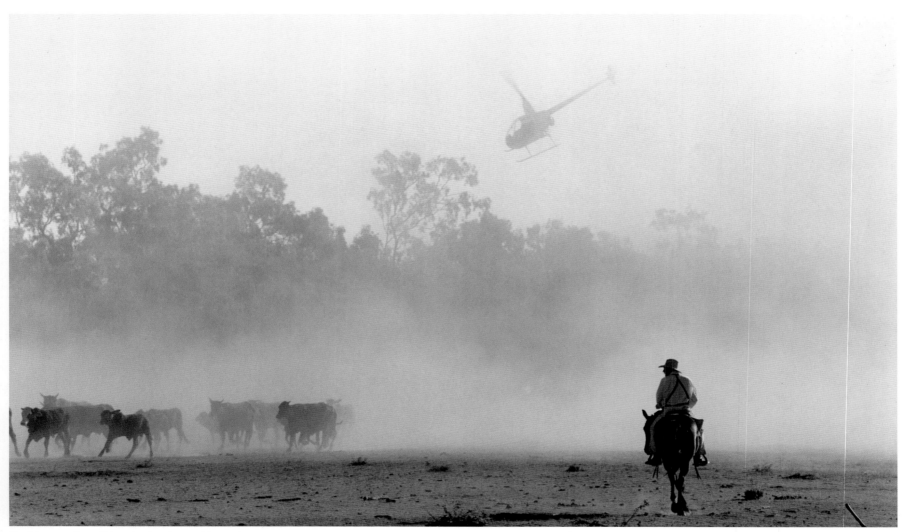

Pushing up the tail late in the day on Vanrook

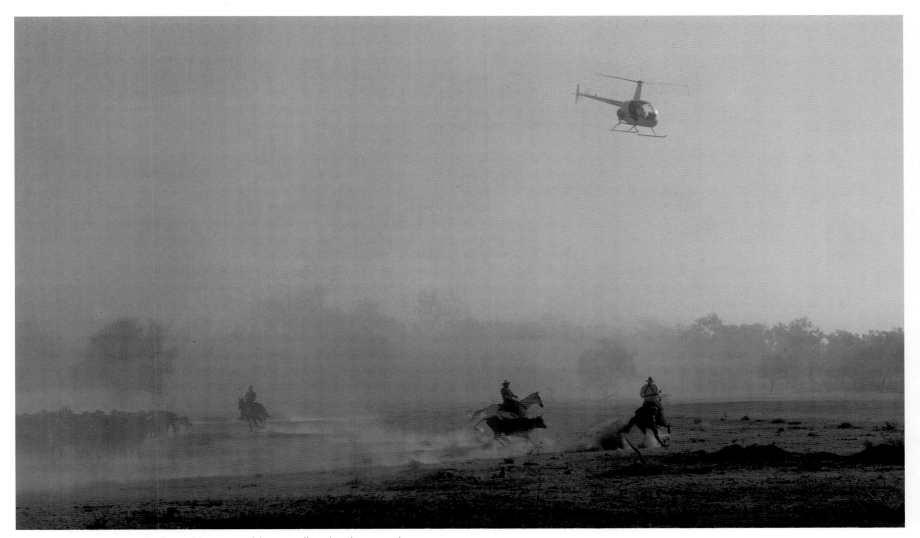

Stockmen and chopper pilot have this wayward beast well and truly covered

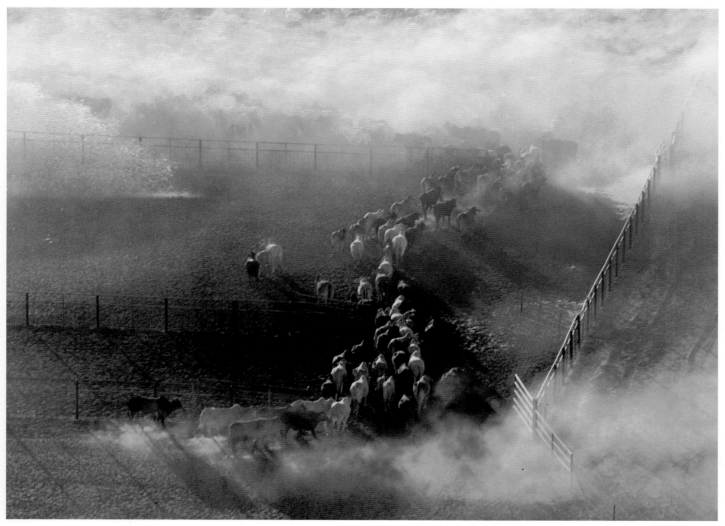

The last of the cattle stream into the yards. The spray to the left of the picture is from a large sprinkler system installed to reduce dust

Facing page: A spectacular sight as over 3000 head crowd into the yards at Keeroongooloo ready for processing the next day

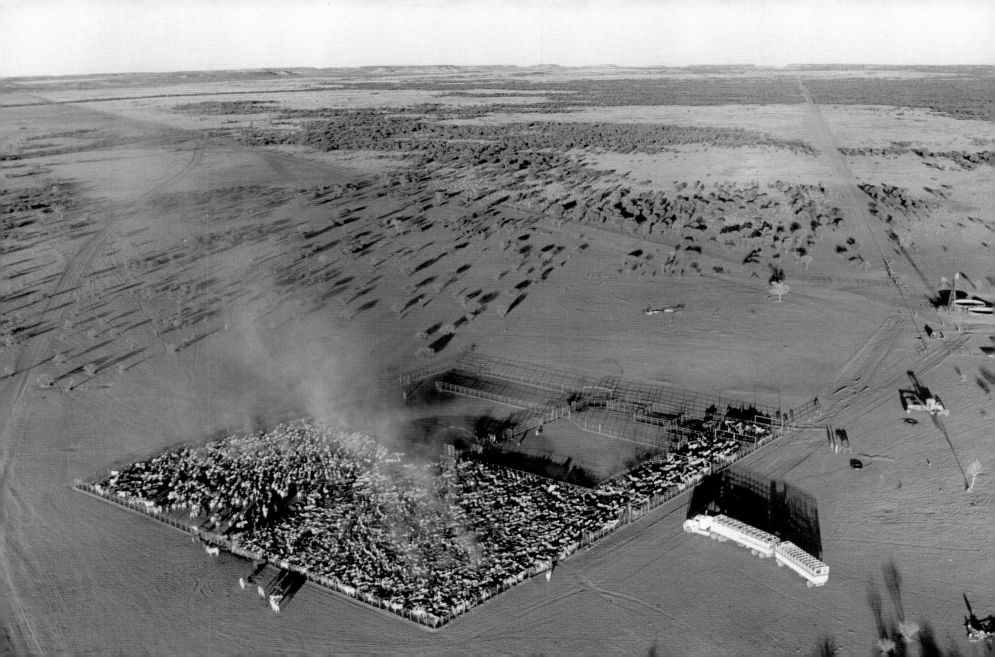

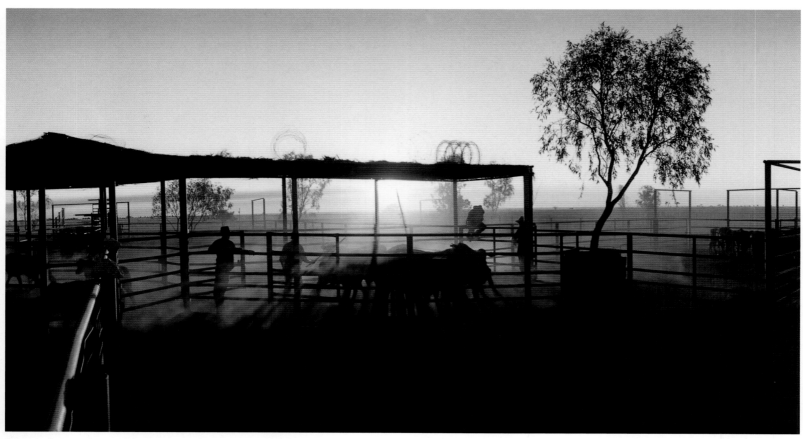

Late drafting at Austral Downs for early morning trucking

Getting the final count before trucking early the following morning at Austral Downs

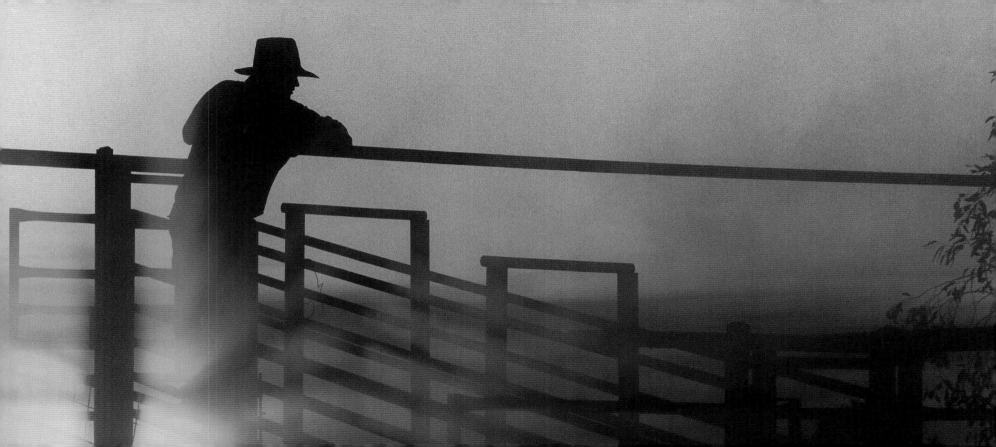

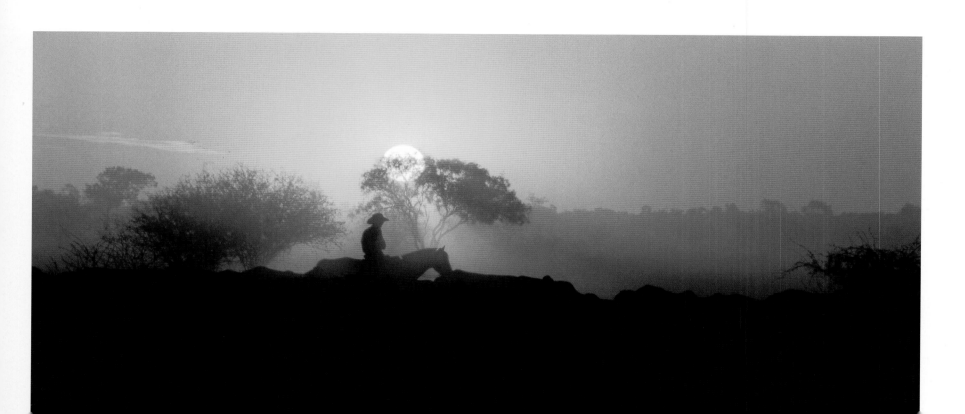

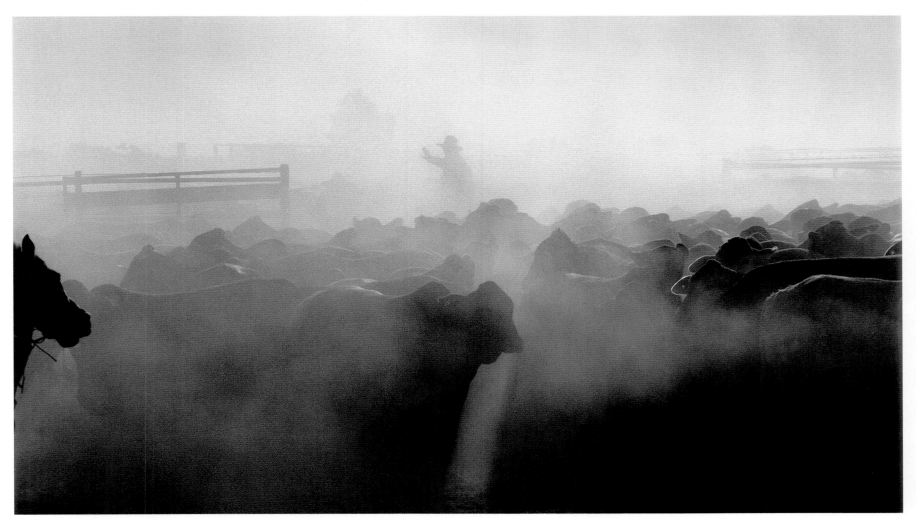

Blocking the gate as they split up the cattle in the Davenport yards to prevent overcrowding

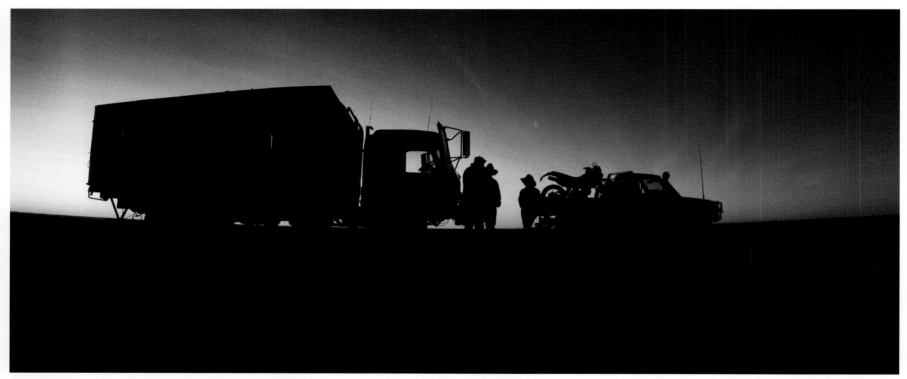

Collecting the truck from where the muster began, as the last rays of light signal the end of the day

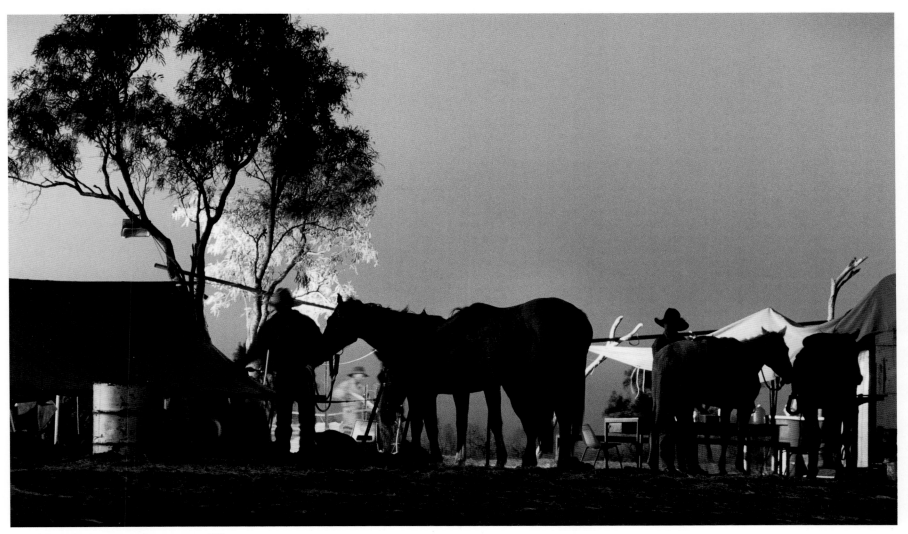

Unsaddling the horses at the camp on Millungera

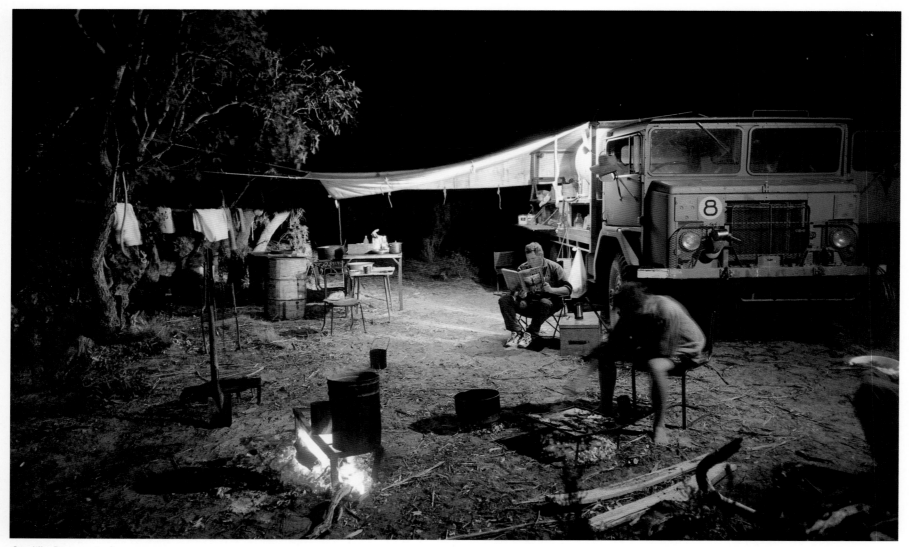

Cordillo Downs stock camp

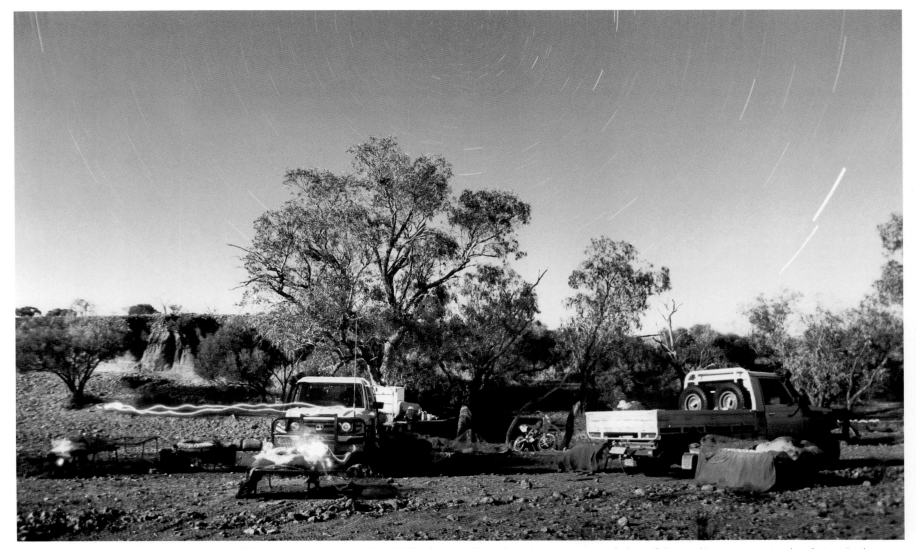

Fast asleep in the camp at Keeroongooloo. (This image was taken in the middle of a moonlit night with an exposure of about 3 hours. You can see streaks of stars in the night sky and what appears to be someone lighting up a smoke, going for a walk and then returning to their swag.)

Photographic Locations

AUSTRAL DOWNS

Austral Downs is owned by the Australian Agricultural Company (AA Company) and is located west of Camoweal in the Northern Territory. It is 526 000 ha (1.3 million acres) and is staffed by 15 full time workers. The property located on the rich Barkly Tablelands runs 20 000 head of Santa Gerturdis cattle and is regarded as one of the AA Companies better breeding properties.

CORDILLO DOWNS

Cordillo Downs is a 809 000 ha (7800 sq. km) property in the top north-eastern corner of South Australia with the Queensland border being the northern and eastern boundaries. It has been owned by the Brook family since 1981.

The property runs around 7000 head of poll hereford cattle and they muster from February through to December. Six men are permanently employed here with mustering done by helicopter, motorbikes and Toyota.

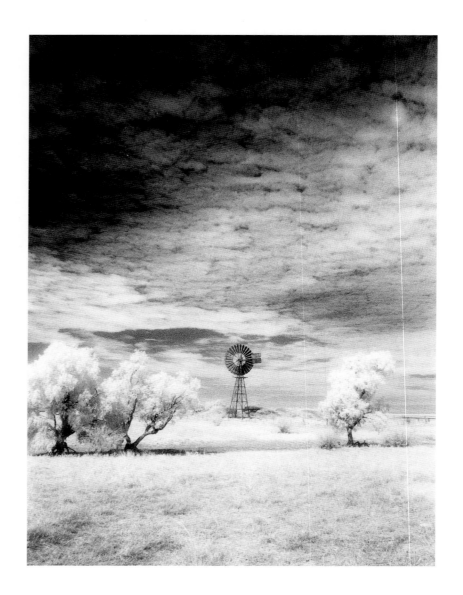

DAVENPORT DOWNS

Owned by the Stanbroke Pastoral Company, Davenport Downs is big by anyones standards. It covers 1.4 million hectares in the Channel Country south-west of Winton. Steers are brought in from the Companies breeding properties on the Barkly Tablelands and the Gulf. The property usually carries around 23 000 head with approximately 10 000 head being turned off each year. Finished cattle are sent direct to meat works all over Queensland and average around 320kg dressed, although those featured in this book averaged about 360kg due to the good season. Davenport Downs has a permanent staff of 16.

KEEROONGOOLOO STATION

Keeroongooloo Station is owned by the Colonial Agricultural Company and covers approximately 607 000 ha (1.5 million acres). The property finishes high grade brahman steers bred on the Companies northern breeding properties. The average size herd on Keeroongooloo is 18 000 head and the property aims to turn off 8000 head every year at an average dressed weight of 310 to 320kg.

There are 8 full time employees with extra help during mustering.

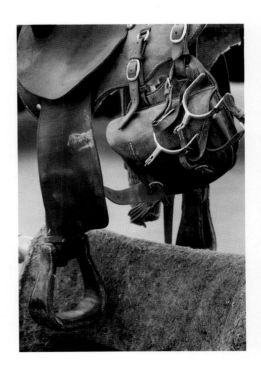

MILLUNGERA STATION

Owned by the Acton Land and Cattle Co. Millungera is situated north of Julia Creek. It covers 364 000 ha (900 000 acres) and carries 30 000 head of cattle consisting of 23 000 Brahman and Santa Gertrudis breeders. The steers are turned off as weaners and sent to either Croydon Station or Moray Downs for finishing. The heifers are either kept for breeding or sent to the Central Queensland finishing properties. There are ususally 25 full time employees on the station and they operate 2 stock camps.

MORAY DOWNS

Moray Downs is west of Clermont in Central Queensland and is also owned by the Acton Land and Cattle Co. and is about 121 500 ha (300 000 acres). It is a finishing property and is located on the Belyando River and comprises mainly buffel grass pastures. It usually runs 22 000 head of Brahman and Santa Gertrudis steers and a number of cull females. Steers are turned off at 24 – 30 months and usually dress around 300kg. There are 6 full time employees on Moray Downs.

TOBERMOREY STATION

A 607 000 ha (1.5 million acre) property just inside the Northern Territory border, west of Urandangi. Although it has since been sold, at the time Tobermorey was owned by the Laglan Pastoral Company and was operated as a commercial breeding and fattening property.

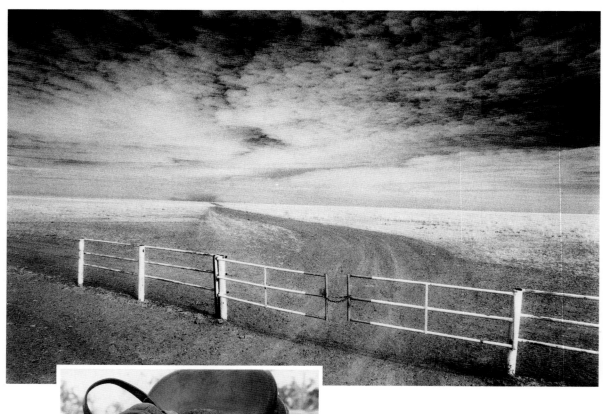

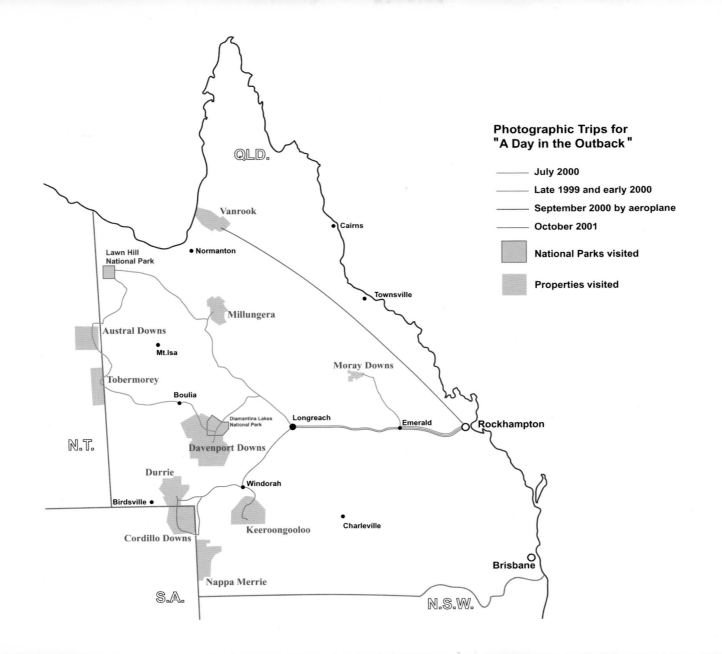

Photographic Trips for "A Day in the Outback"

QLD.

Vanrook

Cairns

Lawn Hill National Park

Normanton

Townsville

Millungera

Austral Downs

Mt.Isa

Moray Downs

Tobermorey

Boulia

Diamantina Lakes National Park

Longreach

Emerald

Rockhampton

N.T.

Davenport Downs

Durrie

Windorah

Birdsville

Keeroongooloo

Charleville

Cordillo Downs

Brisbane

Nappa Merrie

S.A.

N.S.W.

Legend:
- July 2000
- Late 1999 and early 2000
- September 2000 by aeroplane
- October 2001
- National Parks visited
- Properties visited

A DAY IN THE OUTBACK
ISBN 0 9585715 1 1
Pictures and Text: Mark Coombe
© Mark Coombe

First published in 2002 by: Mark Coombe

Many of the images in this book are available as photographic or matt art prints.

For further information contact:
Mark Coombe
Box 5431
Rockhampton
CQMC Queensland 4702 Australia
Ph: 07-49344412
Email: info@markcoombe.com
Website: www.markcoombe.com
Printed in China